KT-481-373

Overcoming Common Problems

Coping with Postnatal Depression

Dr Sandra L. Wheatley

sheldon PRESS

First published in Great Britain in 2005

Sheldon Press
36 Causton Street
London SW1P 4ST

The author and publisher have made every effort to ensure that the external website
and email addresses included in this book are correct and up to date at the time of
going to press. The author and publisher are not responsible for the content, quality
or continuing accessibility of the sites.

British Library Cataloguing-in-Publication Data

A catalogue record for this book is available from the British Library

ISBN 0–85969–930–7

1 3 5 7 9 10 8 6 4 2

Typeset by Deltatype Limited, Birkenhead, Merseyside
Printed in Great Britain by Ashford Colour Press

For the two most recent additions to our family,
Jack and Joceli.

Contents

Introduction

You've recently had a baby and this is probably the last way you expected to feel – weepy, vulnerable, isolated, and perhaps scared to talk to anybody. Now is supposed to be a time for celebration and new life. What could have gone wrong? If you're not feeling as happy as you expected, don't worry – you are not alone. Some one in ten women develop postnatal depression or feelings of sadness and despair after the birth of a baby.

Meet Helen. She took part in the research that formed part of my PhD, and I interviewed her twice, once three months after her son was born and again when he was one year old. Her account of having her son and how her life was changed during this time is in the book *Nine Women, Nine Months, Nine Lives*, the details of which can be found in Further Reading at the back of this book.

Helen was 30 years old when she accidentally became pregnant. She and her husband Richard had been married for six months and had known each other since they were at school. She experienced a great deal of internal conflict about her decision to go ahead with having the baby, having seriously considered a termination well into the first few months of pregnancy, as she had never really seen herself having children. Her husband had always thought he would be a father.

It wasn't until her son was a year old that she confided in me that she thought she had been depressed after Will was born. She described how she had felt trapped at home with the baby and couldn't wait to get back to work. The unrewarding (to her), repetitive tasks involved in caring for a young baby frustrated, irritated and ground her down so much that her confidence in her ability to hold even a simple conversation with other adults took a nosedive. She told me that she had been horrified to realize that she would frequently not speak to her son from the moment he woke up in the morning until well into the afternoon – she just hadn't felt it necessary to interact with him at all. She had to make a conscious effort to speak to him and take an interest in his development.

Before she had Will she thought she was incapable of being a mother. When he was born all the evidence of her own behaviour confirmed to her that that was the case. She did want to be a good mother but felt she didn't even know how to be a good enough mother. From the conversation I had with her three months after Will was born I knew that she wanted to return to work as soon as she could. She emphasized that this was for financial reasons. But underneath what she felt it was acceptable to say even to me, as a psychologist, was the real reason: she really felt it would be for Will's and her own benefit to be apart.

The good news was that this allowed her to retain as much of her sense of self as she could and to be the best mother she could be. Going back to work had helped her to recover from her depression. Naturally I encouraged her to continue getting support from the people she felt she could turn to and soon she was well on the way to feeling better.

The most important thing you can do at the moment, and throughout this very difficult time, is to believe that you will get better. Just like Helen, you really must seek and accept help. Don't delay. Helen regretted not getting help sooner, and felt that she had missed out on an important part of her son's life, one that could never be repeated or replaced.

Many people find it difficult to ask others for help, but it is very important that you do. It is unlikely that your depression will just get better on its own, no matter how much you wish that it would. Please don't feel ashamed of how you are feeling. You are not alone. Always remember that one in ten women who have had a baby feel the way you do. The sooner you get help, the sooner you will be well again. Let that thought give you courage.

Having a baby and becoming a parent is a major event in the lives of women and men. Becoming a parent is usually accompanied by changes to your home life, social life and relationships. Whether this is your first, second or third baby, the first few weeks of parenthood are daunting and demanding, both physically and emotionally.

Popular images of motherhood are often misleading. They suggest that mothers are radiant and energetic, living in perfect homes with supportive partners and happy well-behaved babies and children. Mothering is often believed to be a natural ability that all 'good' women have. You may have expected to love your baby immediately, but this can take a while and it is not always instinctive. Not loving your baby straight away does not mean that you are not a 'good woman' or a 'natural mother'. Becoming a mother can feel like an overwhelming responsibility and it is very easy to feel inadequate when other mothers around you seem to be coping well.

In reality, becoming and being a mother means constantly experiencing new events and carrying out tasks we are not sure we can manage. A new set of skills to cope with these situations have to be learnt, so don't be too hard on yourself. We all learn to be a mother when we actually have a baby, not before. Women do not automatically know how to be a mother. Men do not automatically know how to be a father.

Each woman's experience of having a baby and being a mother is unique. It is likely that during the first few weeks and months of motherhood you will feel a mixture of emotions. Some women feel sad more often than they feel happy. Sometimes this sadness can develop into depression. Women who find the weeks and months after childbirth difficult often imagine that they are the only ones who are not coping. This is simply not true.

If you think you are depressed after your baby is born, please do not despair. In all the years I have been helping women through this difficult time I have never yet met a woman who, after having sought and accepted help, did not recover.

By reading this book you are seeking and accepting help, so I would say that means that you will recover. It will take time and effort, but you will recover. Please believe me.

Postnatal mood changes

Before I go any further I will outline some facts about the mood changes a woman can experience at this time. There are three mood changes that can develop after the birth of a baby: the baby blues, postnatal depression and puerperal psychosis.

The baby blues

The baby blues tend to occur in the first week after delivery and affect as many as eight out of ten of all new mothers. In fact, it is considered usual to experience the blues, even if only for a short while. A woman may burst into tears for no obvious reason, or feel on top of the world one minute and miserable the next. It is quite usual to feel anxious or tense, be lacking in confidence or feel worried.

Postnatal depression

Postnatal depression affects one in ten women following the birth of a baby. This illness usually begins in the first six months after childbirth, although for some women the depression begins in pregnancy. It is important to know that postnatal depression can occur at any time within the first year after the birth of a baby, and can last for longer than a year if help is not sought and received. Untreated postnatal depression can lead to the breakdown of relationships with partners and children.

On an optimistic note, early diagnosis and treatment of postnatal depression will result in a faster recovery. Quite often a close family friend or perhaps the partner of the woman recognizes that she is unwell before the mother realizes it herself.

Puerperal psychosis

Puerperal psychosis is a much rarer and serious mood change, affecting about one in 500 new mothers. The symptoms will appear suddenly, often within the first two weeks following the birth of the baby. Women with a family history of mental illness or who have suffered from puerperal psychosis in the past are at a higher risk of developing this illness.

Symptoms include hallucinations (seeing or hearing things that others cannot), delusions (incredible beliefs such as thinking she can save the world) and mania (extremely energetic and bizarre activity like cleaning the house in the middle of the night). The symptoms can be severe and sometimes very frightening for the woman, her partner and her family. In fact her partner may be the first to realize that she is unwell. So it is important that her partner, or someone close to her, knows the symptoms to look out for.

Medical help should be sought immediately from her GP or from the emergency services. Seeking help quickly will make sure that she is well again quickly. Women with this illness are often treated in hospital and will usually make a full recovery.

The focus of this book

From this point forward I am going to assume that the reader of this book is a woman who has, or thinks she may have, postnatal depression. I will talk to you directly. The main aim of this book is to help you, a woman who has postnatal depression, become well again as quickly as possible. I would also like for you to feel stronger, as an individual, as a result of having survived postnatal depression. This book is here to help you achieve that.

One in ten women who have had a baby has had postnatal depression. Fact. This means that you are not alone. It means that one in ten of the women that you know who have children will understand what you are feeling because they have been depressed too. One in ten of the women at the health visitor's clinic. One in ten of the women at playgroup. One in ten of the women with children at the supermarket. And perhaps most important to remember, as so many of them are women, one in ten of midwives and health visitors who have children. There is no 'us' and 'them' with postnatal depression. It happens to women from all walks of life, regardless of age, culture and social class. One in ten women really means one in ten women.

Talk to someone you can trust about how you are feeling, like your partner, your mum, a friend, or your midwife or health visitor. It can help a lot just to confide in someone else. Once they know how you are feeling they will be able to give you the support you feel you want or need.

Postnatal depression is an illness. It is not your fault you feel the way you do. Please don't be ashamed of how you are feeling. Your midwife, health visitor and GP are all trained to help you. One in ten of them will have personal experience of how you are feeling. They want to help you. So let them try.

You may get on better with one or other of the health professionals involved in your care. Speak to the one you feel you can trust the most. For example, it doesn't matter if now that you have had your baby you don't get on as well with your health visitor as you did with your midwife – if you feel you can be more honest with your midwife then speak to her rather than your health visitor. You will not offend your health visitor. She will be very glad that you have told someone how you feel.

The most important thing you can do is to believe that you will get better, and to seek and accept help. If you haven't already, and you think you are depressed, talk to your midwife, health visitor or GP as soon as you can. By combining their help and this book you really are speeding up your recovery.

Many people find it difficult to ask others for help, but it is very important that you do. It is unlikely that your depression will just get better on its own, no matter how much you wish that it would. You would not expect a broken leg to get better without the help of health professionals. Don't expect your feelings to get better without their help either.

You are only human – you are not perfect. You have limits to what you can do. Each of us can cope with different amounts and types of stress in our lives. You may find yourself asking why you, who previously could cope with working, running a home and having a social life, can no longer seem to cope when working is swapped for motherhood. Simple. Motherhood is a role that contains different types and different amounts of stress. Those differences have led, in part, to your suffering from postnatal depression.

Lack of concentration is a problem for people with depression. And lack of time is a problem for women with young babies and children. This means that a book about postnatal depression needs to be written as simply and concisely as possible. This book is intended to give you information about the emotional changes that can happen after having a baby. This information should help you decide if the emotions you are experiencing after having your baby are usual. If they are not usual then you may want to try some of the suggestions in this book to get you and keep you well. They have worked for many women and so they should work for you too.

This book aims to inform but not overwhelm you. Within each chapter there are several headings so that you can dip in and out of it as you wish. I would recommend starting at the beginning as each chapter builds upon the last, but it has been written so that you will be able to jump between chapters if you want to.

The first couple of chapters focus upon what postnatal depression is, what the symptoms are, which symptoms you have and what the possible causes of your postnatal depression are. Chapters 3 to 6 are for when you can start taking control of your life again. They outline, with simple, practical suggestions, what you can do to help yourself get well, and how you, with help from your partner (if you have one), family and friends, can keep yourself well.

At the back of this book is a list of other books you may like to read and some support groups and organisations for parents, which you might like to contact.

That you are reading this book tells me you want to recover from this illness. You have noticed you have changed and are wondering whether that change has been a good or a bad one. Please don't feel guilty about that change. There seems to be no rhyme or reason why some people get depressed and others don't. The fact is that you are and you want to do something about it. And that is fantastic. Welcome to the road to recovery.

1

How do I know if I am depressed?

Meet Sophie. She is now in her late twenties living in Rutland. She and her partner Darren both worked full-time in London before they decided to start a family. They both wanted to have another child less than a year after their daughter Hannah was born. Soon after their second daughter, Lucy, was born they moved out of London into a house they felt would meet the needs of an expanding young family. They could run their own company from home in an adjoining outbuilding, enabling them to share the care of their offspring. Their lives seemed so well thought out. However, what they hadn't taken into consideration was that while growing up in rural idyll may be wonderful for kids when they are a bit older, it can be very isolating and lonely for a young woman with two children under two years old.

Soon after moving, Sophie remembers relentlessly doing things to distract herself from the emotional void inside her, where she had expected the love for her second daughter to be. She couldn't even muster any affection for her first daughter any more. She felt like a domestic robot. She could keep her house clean, her partner's sexual needs fulfilled, her daughters content and herself well-presented. What she couldn't do was feel anything other than guilt and shame. She couldn't feel happy, she didn't laugh. She did cry, but only when hiding in the bathroom away from anyone who might expect her to be happy. She slept very rarely and lost a great deal of weight. When people expressed concern for her she denied anything was wrong. When she looks back now she thinks she probably wanted to believe that it was just that she was exhausted by her two children and having recently moved house to a new part of the country. So that is what she told herself; she denied even to herself that something was wrong.

Darren was very worried about her, particularly her denial that anything was wrong, and asked his mum for her advice. It took Darren, his mum and Sophie's mum to persuade her to let the doctor come and see her at home, and it took them three long weeks to get her even to consider that what she was feeling was not usual. And yet Sophie says she knew all about postnatal depression. She just never thought it would happen to her.

Symptoms

There are many symptoms of depression; some of the more usual ones are shown below. If you feel any of them *more often than would be usual for you*, please do confide in someone you are able to trust about these feelings. If this person is not your midwife, health visitor or GP then please do talk to them as well, as soon as possible. They will be able to help you get well again. Quite simply, the sooner you ask for help, the sooner you will receive help, feel well and be more able to enjoy your life as a mother.

The symptoms of postnatal depression experienced will be different for each individual. No two women will feel quite the same. You may recognize yourself as having some but not all of the following symptoms. The symptoms can often change over the course of the illness, with some being more problematic earlier on in the illness than others. Again, this pattern will be unique for each woman.

Some of the more usual symptoms of postnatal depression

A woman with postnatal depression may:

- *Be anxious and fearful.* You may feel very anxious; you may become obsessed with unjustified fears about your baby, yourself or your partner. You may only feel safe if someone is with you all the time, feeling fearful of being left alone with the baby. You may have overwhelming fears about, for example, you or the baby dying.
- *Worry a lot.* Unjustified worries about things you normally take for granted. It is important to remember that everybody worries from time to time, but when does worrying become too much worrying? Answer: when it is more than would be usual for you.
- *Have uncontrollable feelings of panic.* This is when your heart beats faster, the palms of your hands become sweaty and you may feel sick, even that you are going to faint. These attacks can occur

at any time, but they are most common in new or stressful situations.

- *Feel tense.* Your neck and shoulders may feel tight and you may be unable to unwind and relax, even when you try. In fact you may find that the harder you try to relax, the more tense you feel.
- *Have more physical aches and pains.* These can include headaches, blurred vision and stomach pains. These may be signs of tension and your body's way of telling you you are unwell.
- *Be irritable.* For no good reason you may find yourself shouting and snapping at your baby or your children, your partner or others who cannot understand what they have done to deserve your anger.
- *Feel sad.* This can vary from just feeling low, to utter despair, as if your world is an empty place. Your thoughts are negative and focus on your failures. You might even feel that your baby or partner would be better off without you.
- *Cry a lot or feel tearful.* Although some women may not actually cry, they describe feeling that they are often on the verge of crying. Or you may weep steadily for entire days.
- *Feel less hungry.* Not feeling hungry, not wanting to eat as much as usual, or even not eating at all. This can lead to extreme weight loss.
- *Feel more hungry.* Alternatively you may comfort eat as a way of coping with your feelings of depression. This may lead to extreme weight gain.
- *Be unable to sleep.* You may have difficulty sleeping, either not being able to get off to sleep, or waking up very early and not going back to sleep. This can be particularly frustrating when you cannot sleep even when your baby is sleeping soundly.
- *Sleep a lot.* Alternatively some women describe wanting to sleep all the time, no matter how much sleep they have had – this is not just due to the sleepless nights that all new parents experience.
- *Feel exhausted.* You may feel constantly tired, lethargic and drained of energy, so much so that you feel unable to cope with daily tasks.
- *Be unable to concentrate.* You may feel easily distracted and confused, finding it difficult to finish tasks that you start, like the washing, reading a magazine or watching TV.
- *Be unable to make decisions.* Making simple decisions such as what to wear may seem impossible. You may spend a lot of time

3

making lists in an attempt to get organized but never decide when or how you are going to do the things on your lists.

- *Feel unable to cope.* Even simple everyday things, things you used to do without even thinking about, are beyond you. Because you are having to try so hard to do even the little things to get by, you may feel inadequate and incapable, and start questioning your ability to look after your baby completely.

- *Take little interest in your appearance and surroundings.* You don't see the point in washing yourself or getting dressed, and have no interest in your home or your everyday life.

- *Take too much interest in your appearance and surroundings.* Alternatively you may become obsessively tidy and try to maintain impossibly high standards in the home.

- *Feel hopeless.* Being unable to look forward to things in general any more, you may feel that there is no point in trying to do anything, that life and everything in it is hopeless.

- *Feel a loss of pleasure in activities usually enjoyed.* For example, going out with friends might seem difficult, and you may even find just talking to people is too much for you.

- *Feel no interest in sex.* Many women find that they are not interested in sex for a while after their baby is born. They may need time to heal after the birth, and may be too tired in those early weeks and months of being a mother. However, with postnatal depression it may take a lot longer to regain an interest in a sexual relationship. This can become another source of stress, which can be very difficult for both you and your partner.

- *Feel guilty.* One of the many emotions women describe is an overwhelming sense of guilt. You may feel that you should be 'grateful for your beautiful baby', or perhaps you feel guilty about not being the wonderful mother you hoped you would be.

- *Feel ashamed.* Feeling ashamed about not being able to 'pull yourself together' can lead to you blaming yourself. Often it is difficult to admit to feeling this way even to yourself.

- *Think strange thoughts.* For example, you may believe that by not walking on the cracks in the pavement, your baby will sleep through the night, or you may be convinced that if you *do* walk on the cracks in the pavement, your baby will die. Some depressed mothers may have recurrent thoughts about harming their baby. These thoughts can be very frightening and cause you very real distress.

4

Identifying postnatal depression

To help find out if you are feeling depressed, it is likely that your health visitor will ask you to fill in a questionnaire about six weeks after the birth. It is called the *Edinburgh Postnatal Depression Scale* which was developed in 1987 by John Cox (a psychiatrist), Jenny Holden (a health visitor) and Ruth Sagovsky (a researcher). It consists of ten simple questions. Your health visitor will be using her clinical judgement (her years of training and experience) in combination with this questionnaire to try to see if you are vulnerable to suffering from postnatal depression. The maximum score is 30; a score of 12 or more would tell her that you are.

Please be honest with yourself and with them when completing that questionnaire. Remember that it is an illness. It is not your fault you feel the way that you do. Your midwife, health visitor and GP are all trained to help you. One in ten of them will have personal experience of how you are feeling. They want to help you. So help them to help you by being honest.

You may have already completed the Edinburgh Postnatal Depression Scale. If so, and you scored 12 or more, your health visitor has probably offered to come and see you at home to talk about how you are feeling. Many health visitors call these 'listening visits', as their main aim is to listen to you talk about how you are feeling. They may also make suggestions about ways of coping with things that are bothering you, and about support groups that you could go along to. Your health visitor may be interested to know that you are reading this book, so show it to her when next you see her. She will know, just as I do, that wanting to help yourself is a very positive first step on the road to recovery.

Your health visitor may also have recommended that you go and see your GP to talk about how you are feeling. They will be able to offer you forms of treatment that your health visitor cannot, including referral to counsellors or therapists, and perhaps anti-depressant medication. The many different options for treatment available to you will be discussed in more detail in Chapter 3. Try to keep an open mind about who can help you become well again. Don't decide not to go and see your GP because you think she might want to prescribe you antidepressants, if you don't want to take them. She will be able to offer you other forms of help, which you may find more acceptable.

If your health visitor hasn't asked you to complete the Edinburgh Postnatal Depression Scale, or you would simply like to know how you are feeling at the moment, you can complete the questionnaire below.

The Four-Weekly Wheatley Questionnaire

This questionnaire aims to compare how you usually feel with how you have been feeling recently. What I mean by how you usually feel is how you felt in general before you became pregnant with your (most recent) baby.

Please think back to the months before you became pregnant. Take a few moments to remember how you would generally feel in your everyday life. For example, how you felt about work (if you were working), how you felt about your partner (if you have one), and how you felt about yourself – your abilities, your confidence, and your contentment with your life. It will help you to think about this if you stop reading, look up from the page and gaze into space for a moment or two.

Done that? Good. Now think about how you have been feeling in the past week. It is very important that you think back over the whole of the past week so that your answers to the questions reflect how you have been feeling recently rather than just how you have been feeling today. This is especially important if today has been a day when you have been feeling very unwell, or on the other hand, very well.

For example, if today is a Monday, think back to what you were doing last Monday. Then spend a few moments just thinking about what you have done and what has happened on the days between then and now. Please spend another few moments thinking about *how you felt* about the things you have done and what has happened since then. As before, it will help you to think about this if you stop reading and look up from the page and gaze into space for a moment or two.

Done that as well? Good. Now fill in the questionnaire, comparing how you usually feel with how you have felt in the past week. Tick one of the boxes to show whether or not you have felt that way *in general* in the past week. Please be honest with yourself.

HOW DO I KNOW IF I AM DEPRESSED?

The Four-Weekly Wheatley Questionnaire*

		Yes	No
1	Have you felt tired more than is usual for you?		
2	Have you been feeling more irritable than is usual for you?		
3	Have you felt less hungry than is usual for you?		
4	Have you been feeling less energetic than is usual for you?		
5	Have you been feeling sad more than is usual for you?		
6	Have you been worrying more than is usual for you?		
7	Have you been crying more than is usual for you?		
8	Have you been unable to look forward to things more than is usual for you?		
9	Have you felt unable to cope with everyday tasks more than is usual for you?		
10	Have you felt guilty more than is usual for you?		
	Total:		

* © Potent 2004

Now add up the number of 'Yes' and 'No' boxes you have ticked and write that in the total box (10 is the maximum you can score).

The total number of 'Yes' answers you gave is the score referred to below. The number of 'Yes' boxes you ticked shows just how postnatally depressed you may or may not be.

What your score means

• A score of 0: This shows that you have not been postnatally depressed in the past week.
• A score between 1 and 3: This shows that you are likely to have been feeling mildly postnatally depressed in the past week.
• A score between 4 and 6: This shows that you are likely to have been feeling moderately or really quite postnatally depressed in the past week.
• A score between 7 and 10: This shows that you are likely to have been feeling severely or very postnatally depressed in the past week.

Asking for and getting help

If your answers to the questionnaire show that you are likely to be postnatally depressed at the moment, even if only mildly, then you should talk to your midwife, health visitor or GP as soon as you can. Speak to whichever one of them you feel you can trust.

If your answers show that you are likely to be severely or very postnatally depressed then it is extremely important to talk to a health professional immediately. Telephone them and arrange an appointment as soon as you possibly can. You are unwell and need help. They will be able to help you.

As well as speaking to a health professional about how you are feeling, it would be a good idea to talk to someone close to you, like your mum, your partner, a friend, or another relative like a sister or your grandmother.

If you do not feel able to cope with explaining how you feel to a health professional on your own, ask someone that you trust to be with you – again, perhaps your partner, your mum, or a friend. Or you could ask your midwife, health visitor or GP to come and see you at home if you prefer.

Once you have got in place the help you feel suits you, you can monitor how you are feeling by completing the questionnaire again in four weeks' time. I would recommend repeating the exercise once a month for as long as you feel you want or need to. It is important to wait about a month after you have completed it the first time to give time for the help you have sought and accepted to have a noticeable positive impact on your illness.

By doing this once a month you will be able to share with your health visitor, partner and/or mum how your illness is responding to the help you have been offered and received. Hopefully you will see that the way you are feeling is changing for the better. This should give you a real boost, and encourage you to keep accepting the support you are being offered. It will also encourage you to keep on helping yourself, as outlined in Chapters 4 and 5.

If the next time you complete the questionnaire there is no change in your score, you may want to consider reviewing the amount and type of support you are accepting; or you may equally want to give it another month and see what your score reveals then about how much the support you are receiving is helping you. It is really up to you. Talk about it with your health visitor, partner and/or mum. Remember that when speaking to a health professional no question is ever too small or silly. If you want to know the answer, just ask.

If your score increases at any time, indicating that your depression is increasing, it is extremely important to talk to someone immediately. Get in touch with the health professional you trust and arrange an appointment with them, either for you to go and see them, or for them to come and see you, as soon as you possibly can. You will need to review the amount and type of support you are accepting as the increase in your score shows that it isn't having the desired positive effect.

Completing this questionnaire on a regular monthly basis cannot do you any harm. Looking on the bright side, your score on the questionnaire will result in one of the following three scenarios: either you will be able to see how much you are getting better; or you will be able to see how much you are not getting worse; or last, and perhaps most important, you will get an early warning that you need more, and perhaps a different type of, support.

What you can do now

To tide you over until you come to the later chapters in this book about how to help yourself to recover from this illness, take a moment to think about what you could do after you have finished this chapter that would make you feel a bit better. Something that will make you feel like you are making a start. For example, other women have found it helps them to sit still for a while and think about what they have just read and what it has helped them to learn about themselves: how depressed they are, how much courage it took to fill in the questionnaire honestly, who they think they could share that information with, and what they think those people's reaction to that conversation will be. Perhaps while you are sitting there contemplating these thoughts, you could put your feet up and have a rest for a few moments. You might prefer to get out of the house and go for a walk to try to take in what you have read and what you have realized. You might like to telephone a friend and chat about how you are feeling. Whatever you think will help you to take in the information you have just read, do it. It will help you to start to take control of how you feel and what you think. It will help you to believe you will get better.

As I said before, the most important thing you can do at the moment, and throughout this very difficult time, is to believe that you will get better. You must seek and accept help. Many people find it difficult to ask for help but it is very important that you do. It is unlikely that your depression will just get better on its own, no matter how much you wish that it would.

Please don't feel ashamed of how you are feeling. You are not alone. Always remember that one in ten women who have had a baby feel the way you do. The sooner you get help, the sooner you will be well again. Let that thought give you courage.

2

Why me?

Why am I feeling depressed?

There are various reasons why you might be feeling depressed – or a combination of reasons. The main thing to remember is that it isn't your fault, and that no matter what the reason, there is a way forward.

Women are at greater risk of suffering from depression

In general, women are between two and three times more at risk of developing depression than men. Three explanations for why this is the case are widely accepted, and they are biological, psychological and sociological in basis. That is, although there are exceptions, it is widely believed that men and women differ from each other in these three areas.

There are the obvious biological differences between us, for example in our genes and in our hormones. There are also noted psychological differences between men and women, such as the way women value social contact with others much more so than men. Finally, we are all influenced by society and the stereotypical behaviours expected of women and men; it is thus generally believed that women are more nurturing and caring than men and so are 'naturally' better at parenting.

It is thought that one or other of these differences may explain why women are more likely to get depressed than men. In reality it is probably a combination of two or maybe all three areas of difference.

How does postnatal depression differ from depression?

There has been much debate among academics and clinicians as to whether postnatal depression is a separate illness from a depression that occurs at any other time in our lives. The symptoms of postnatal depression can differ from those of depression at other times in that they almost always include physical symptoms, which do not necessarily occur with depression. The basic difference is that the depression has to occur in the first year after childbirth for it to be called postnatal depression. For a clinical diagnosis of postnatal depression to be made you have to be a woman and you have to have had a baby.

Can men develop postnatal depression?

Men can and do get depressed in the first year after the birth of a child. Partners of women who develop postnatal depression are under great additional pressure to cope – they often take over some or all of the care of the baby, while trying to care for their ill partner, and cope with going to work as well. In fact they are doing all the things and more besides that led to their wife or girlfriend to get depressed in the first place. So logically those men are more vulnerable than the partners of women who have not developed the illness.

The question of whether a man can suffer from postnatal depression is simple. Using the definition of the depression having to occur in the first year after childbirth, then yes it can be said that men can develop postnatal depression too. Naturally the criteria for clinical diagnosis cannot be met as he is not a woman. But whatever words are used to label the way a man is feeling, the fact remains that he is not feeling great. If he is depressed he needs to get some help. Frankly, if the doctor called it loobble disease it wouldn't matter – what matters is that he gets help to relieve the symptoms he is feeling.

What is important is that if a new father suspects he may be feeling depressed he should not worry about what it is called, but seek and accept help from people he trusts in exactly the same way as I outline for mothers in this book. If you think your partner is feeling strained and stressed out more than would be usual for him, get him to fill in the questionnaire in the previous chapter. If he is depressed then it would be a good idea for him to read through this book as well, and then together you can try and help yourselves and each other.

The causes of postnatal depression

Depression is generally divided up into two categories, being either organic or reactive in causation. 'Organic' refers to the physical body and the organ affected by the illness, and in the case of depression that is the brain. 'Reactive' refers to the mind's mental or psychological reaction to circumstances and life events.

The brain is the organ that, if you like, contains the mind. It is an organ just like your heart. When you have an illness that affects your heart you can experience physical symptoms like chest pain. When you have an illness that affects your brain you can experience mental symptoms like depression.

The causes of, or reasons for, postnatal depression can also be separated into organic or reactive, physical or mental. This book focuses on the more common reactive or mental type of depression.

A large amount of research has shown that there are many possible causes of postnatal depression. It can be useful to know what may have triggered your particular postnatal depression, especially if it was a mental or psychological reaction to social circumstances. That way you can try and minimize wherever possible, and preferably avoid, the negative impact of any future situations like the one that triggered this depression.

Everyone is different, and the possible reason or combination of reasons for your depression will be unique to yourself, both physically and mentally as an individual, and your life situation and circumstances. Some of the potential causes of postnatal depression are listed below. You will probably recognize some of them as being potential causes of your own postnatal depression.

Physical causes: an organic reaction to bodily imbalance

It is important to note that the symptoms of some physical illnesses can overlap with the symptoms of mental illness. For instance, you may think the depression is causing your symptoms of, say, sleepiness, weepiness, irritability and loss of appetite, whereas in fact you could be suffering from *hypothyroidism* (your thyroid gland is producing too little of the hormone thyroxin).

This would really be quite rare, but it would be best to speak to your GP to have other causes of your symptoms ruled out. These might include *anaemia, vitamin deficiency* (for example B12), *interactions between and/or side effects from medications* and, as mentioned above, *problems with your thyroid*. A small number of women who develop postnatal depression do have a temporary thyroid gland defect. Once the hypothyroidism has been treated, their depression lifts.

The impact of hormones, specifically the *reproductive hormones* of oestrogen and progesterone, may be a potential cause to explore, particularly if you suffer from premenstrual syndrome and so may

13

already have an imbalance of reproductive hormones. I have included in Further Reading a book by Katharina Dalton called *Depression After Childbirth: How to Recognize, Treat, and Prevent Postnatal Depression*, which approaches postnatal depression as an illness caused by hormonal imbalance. However, the evidence for the role of reproductive hormones in the cause of postnatal depression, as outlined in this book, first published two decades ago, has never been proven. Call me a cynic if you like, but if the only cause of postnatal depression was hormones, a pharmaceutical company would have developed a 'postnatal depression pill' to cure us all by now. They would have made a fortune and I would be out of a job.

So, although progesterone is sometimes used for prevention or treatment, its effectiveness is still uncertain. Any positive results from research into the treatment of postnatal depression by progesterone therapy are equally likely to be attributable to a placebo effect, that is, the increased contact with a health professional, rather than any actual effect of the hormone. An imbalance in reproductive hormones is only one possible cause, and a pretty unlikely one at that. So much so that many midwives and GPs do not recommend hormone therapy.

A *previous personal experience of depression* or a *family history of depression* can be an indicator that a person is at increased risk of developing depression. This is perhaps the most predictable factor in the development of postnatal depression, as around one in two women who have had the illness in the past are at risk of suffering again.

If you were *feeling depressed in your pregnancy* (*antenatal depression*), you are likely to be at a greater risk of developing postnatal depression. You are probably twice as likely as the average woman to suffer the illness.

There is robust evidence for the predictive relationship between previous personal experience of depression, a family history of depression and feeling depressed in your pregnancy, unlike for hormones, and the risk represented by these three factors is addressed as a matter of routine by health professionals involved in your care. It is quite probable that your midwife asked you whether you or anyone in your family had had depression in the past when she did your antenatal booking at the beginning of your pregnancy. This was because she knew that if that was the case you might have benefited from some additional support from her. Throughout your pregnancy she will have asked you how you are feeling, hopefully encouraging you to talk about your feelings as well as your backache!

If you were feeling down in your pregnancy, and you had talked about this with her, she would have passed that information on to your health visitor, so that your health visitor would know that you had had antenatal depression. She would then offer you some additional support after the baby was born to try and prevent you developing, or at the very least reduce the impact of, postnatal depression.

The support that is available from health professionals, and which could usefully be offered by others you trust, will be outlined in more detail in Chapter 3.

Mental causes: a psychological reaction to social circumstances

The interaction between your personal situation and your ability, or rather your inability, to cope with that situation can lead to you feeling depressed.

Unsurprisingly, social factors such as poverty, inappropriate or unsuitable housing, unemployment and being a refugee or asylum-seeker will all contribute to making depression more likely. A new mother is more likely to be depressed if she has experienced recent stressful events in her life – a serious illness, domestic violence or bereavement, for example. Having a number of young children already, expecting twins, feeling unsure about the pregnancy, having a traumatic or difficult birth, or a premature or unwell baby, are also sometimes associated with postnatal depression. The following are various mental factors that are commonly associated with postnatal depression.

Individual differences

Each of us has our own unique personality. We all cope with stressful situations differently and our ability to cope with them changes over our lifetime as we experience more of life. Likewise, we each adapt to new situations differently and have differing attitudes towards change. Some of us welcome new situations and thrive on change, but most of us feel uneasy, nervous or hesitant and just hope that the first time we do something new we don't make too much of a mess of it. Particularly if that doing something new is being a mother. And there are a lot of things to do for the first time when you are a mum. In fact, in the early days there will be something you haven't done before nearly every day. That is an awful lot of anxiety to deal with. This can contribute to the development of postnatal depression.

Homosexuality, and in this context, more specifically how a woman copes with her homosexuality when becoming a mother, is another aspect of individual difference that can impact on her mental health.

> Meet Moira. She was one half of a lesbian couple I worked with. They had decided they wanted to start a family and took it in turns to get pregnant, using the same donor father. Moira's partner Alison was the first to have a baby. Alison was confident in her sexuality and the way she lived her life, and rationalized that her baby would be better off than many, having two mothers and one father. However, when Moira had her baby she found the experience of giving birth very traumatic (she had an emergency caesarean section). In addition she found that having two such small babies to look after between them (there was less than six months between their sons) made life almost unbearably manic. But what she described as the straw that broke the camel's back was the way she felt other people (including their own families) viewed their decision to start a family. She developed postnatal depression about two months after her son was born. Her limited ability to cope with this aspect of her life wasn't the only cause of the depression for her, but it certainly contributed to it.

If this is an issue for you or someone you know, contact PACE (promoting lesbian and gay health and well-being) for information and support; the number is listed in Useful Addresses.

Fertility problems

Wanting to have a child and not being able to can feel like a terrible curse. The medical involvement and depersonalizing techniques of hormone therapy and IVF can seem never-ending. For so long, the daily focus of your thoughts has been on how wonderful your life will be when you finally have a baby. You have spent so long trying to get pregnant that when you finally do, it comes as a huge relief. However, there often follows a very anxious nine months while you worry about whether everything will be all right. If you have not been realistic in your expectations of motherhood, it is possible you will become depressed. As you have had so long to fantasize about having a baby, the not-so-perfect reality of being a mother can come as a disappointment. Also, successful fertility treatment can result in twins or a multiple birth, which is a further risk factor.

Twins and multiple births

If having one baby dependent on you for everything except oxygen for 24 hours a day doesn't sound too daunting, how about two or three babies? The sheer physical energy required to carry, give birth to and then bring up twins, triplets or more would qualify most of us as Olympic athletes. The mental capacity required is phenomenal. I know: I have younger twin brothers and I still don't know to this day how my mum managed. So, unsurprisingly, having more than one baby from one pregnancy is a risk factor for postnatal depression. You can contact the Twins And Multiple Births Association (TAMBA) for support – see Useful Addresses.

Termination

Women who have had a termination in the past can, in subsequent pregnancies, feel guilty about the baby they didn't have, even if they still believe it was the right thing to do at the time. This shame and guilt can result in them feeling depressed during their pregnancy and after they have had the baby.

Miscarriage

Women who have had a miscarriage in the past are likely, in subsequent pregnancies, to feel very anxious about the baby they are currently having. A history of multiple miscarriages will obviously make them even more anxious. This anxiety often peaks around the time they previously miscarried; after this time they may then begin to relax and enjoy their pregnancy. If, however, this heightened antenatal anxiety does not subside, it can become a contributing factor for postnatal depression. You can contact Babyloss for support and counselling – see Useful Addresses.

Stillbirth

As for termination and miscarriage, women who have had a stillbirth in the past may feel very anxious about the baby they are currently having. This anxiety will obviously be more likely to peak towards the end of the pregnancy, around the time of the previous stillbirth, which means therefore that they may be anxious throughout their entire pregnancy. This heightened and protracted period of antenatal anxiety can become a contributing factor for postnatal depression. You can contact SANDS, the Stillbirth and Neonatal Death Society, for support and counselling – see Useful Addresses.

Unwanted pregnancy

An unplanned pregnancy is not necessarily an unwanted pregnancy. As many as seven out of ten pregnancies are unplanned. I wouldn't be here if my conception had been planned. Unfortunately some women who find themselves unexpectedly pregnant really do not want to have the baby. They may have suffered rape or sexual abuse. They may have felt that their family was complete and did not want any more children. Whatever the reason, the fact that the pregnancy is unwanted puts the woman under an enormous amount of emotional strain. This can lead to feelings of depression.

Difficult pregnancy

The pregnancy may be physically very uncomfortable, there may be obstetric complications, you may feel revulsion at your changing body shape, and feel extremely frustrated at being so immobile. All these aspects should resolve themselves after the baby is born; however, a pregnancy spent feeling mentally uncomfortable for physical reasons may increase the likelihood of postnatal depression occurring, particularly if further problems of one kind or another develop after the baby is born.

Difficult or traumatic birth

The feeling that a birth was difficult or traumatic is personal to each individual woman. Put a different woman through the same birth and she will react to it differently, perceiving it as more or less difficult. All our perceptions are relative to our expectations and our previous experiences. For example, as I report in my book *Nine Women, Nine Months, Nine Lives*, for some women having a caesarean section was not so traumatic, as they were terrified of a vaginal delivery. Their perception was that a caesarean section would be preferable to a vaginal delivery and so were relieved when they were offered one – even when it was an emergency. A difficult birth can sometimes result in the illness of the baby, particularly if the baby is born too soon. You can contact the Birth Crisis Network and Bliss for support and counselling – see Useful Addresses.

Unrealistic expectations of what it is like to be a parent

Some women may find that the reality of life as an expectant or new mother is very different from how they had imagined it to be. Much of our conception of being a mother comes from society and the media and the image portrayed of motherhood is usually an overwhelmingly positive one. However, this is not a realistic image, and if we believe it we will be disappointed. This feeling of being let down can be the cause of depression. Aspiring to perfection is not a bad thing, of course, as long as we accept that none of us is perfect, nor are we likely to achieve perfection.

Loss of independence

'Life will never be the same again.' The birth of a baby brings permanent changes to a new mother's life. Babies are hard work, with the constant tasks of feeding, bathing, comforting their crying, and putting them to sleep. The new mother is suddenly responsible, 24 hours a day. A new mother loses the freedom she had before the baby was born. Postnatal depression is potentially an adjustment to loss. Your depression may be a grieving process for the loss of your old self, your old life, your old freedom and independence. This can also be the case with a second or subsequent baby, as your life changes every time you have a baby.

Loss of status

Most women work nowadays, and if you do not return to work after having a baby the lowly status of 'motherhood' in society is likely to come as a disappointment. Particularly when you consider the amount of sheer hard work involved in being a mother. Social roles have a strong link to our self-esteem, and if we feel that our role in society is not highly valued, then our self-esteem will suffer. This increases the likelihood that we will become depressed. As a pregnant woman you had status. However, you will have noticed that the public's attention was transferred from you to the baby very swiftly after the birth. You may wonder whether the care and concern people had for you while you were pregnant was actually directed at the baby, not you – you just happened to be the incubator.

19

WHY ME?

This is highly unlikely to be the case, but feeling this way can make postnatal depression a real possibility.

Isolation

Women who feel isolated, separated from their families or without a supportive partner, can be more likely to suffer from postnatal depression. If you previously worked, you may find that the lack of contact with colleagues, no matter how small and seemingly insignificant, may lead to feelings of intense loneliness. However, it is not necessary to be alone to feel lonely. A woman living in a house with her partner, toddler, mother-in-law and father-in-law can still feel that she has no one to confide in. Throughout this book I repeat endlessly how important it is to talk to someone you can trust about how you feel. If you feel there is no one in your personal life who fits that role, always remember that the health professionals are there for you to turn to, and organizations such as Home-Start have befriending schemes that you could benefit from. Home-Start's contact details are listed in Useful Addresses.

Cultural expectations

Within some cultures there is still a great deal of pressure for women to have sons. I once witnessed a woman who had a baby girl be commiserated with, and wished better luck next time, by an aunt. Many women have told me of similar experiences. Second-generation British-Asian women sometimes feel a conflict between the way they were raised (in Britain as independent individuals within an equal opportunity society) and the more traditional way they are expected to behave once they are married and have a family. Traditions such as a six-week period of 'lying in' can be positive if the woman is encouraged to rest, and if she actually wants to rest. European women might view these traditions wistfully, but I'm sure that not being able to go out of the house at all could get a bit tiresome before the six weeks are up.

Sometimes the help offered by extended family members is well-intentioned but can feel like interference. The physical closeness of living with relatives might put the mother and her relationship with her partner under considerable strain. All these factors add up and can result in a woman feeling depressed after having a baby. The additional unfortunate fact here is that the stigma associated with mental illness, while being bad enough in white European culture, is often much worse in other cultures. Whatever the culture, this stigma all too often results in women not seeking help quickly, for fear of bringing shame on themselves and their family. The fear of their family's negative reaction to their illness only compounds their feelings of hopelessness and exacerbates their depression.

Relationship changes

The birth of a child will have an impact on all your close relationships. If this is your first baby, your own mother will now be a grandmother and your partner now the father of your child. Your beliefs about how a 'grandmother' or a 'father' should behave may conflict with how others react to the new situation, and this may put your relationships under an enormous strain. Various organizations can help with lists of relationship counsellors, and/or contact Relate for support and counselling – see Useful Addresses.

The death of someone close to you

The loss of a loved one, be it recent or some time before, may be brought into sharp relief with the birth of a baby. The deceased may have been someone you felt you wanted to share the birth of your baby with and rely upon for support – your father, a sister, a friend. There is overwhelming evidence to show that losing your mother at an early age makes you more likely to suffer depression. Obviously, the death of someone close to you is likely to make you feel sad, and this in combination with the birth of a baby can increase the risk of developing postnatal depression. You can contact CRUSE for support and counselling – see Useful Addresses.

The illness of someone close to you

Likewise, the illness of someone close to you, with all the worry this brings, will take its toll, all the more so if you are involved in the day-to-day practical care of the person. This constant anxiety and extra physical effort may well lead to exhaustion and contribute to postnatal depression if you, as the carer, do not have, or do not allow, others to care for you. You can contact Carers UK for support and counselling – see Useful Addresses.

Financial worries

If you or your partner loses your job, you could have not only financial but housing worries. You and your family may be threatened with loss of earnings and also with being homeless.

Neither of these situations is likely to enhance your life at any time, and least of all when you are expecting or have recently had a baby. Obviously, these factors would exacerbate the risk of postnatal depression. You can contact the National Debt Helpline and the Maternity Alliance for more information – see Useful Addresses.

Experiencing violence in the home

Domestic violence can be defined as the mental, sexual or physical abuse of a person, committed by any member of their household. This includes partners, stepchildren, mothers-in-law. Domestic violence often raises a number of concerns in a woman's mind. If she is currently being abused, she may wonder how she will be able to prevent the baby witnessing the violence, or indeed how she can protect the baby from her abuser. A very stressful situation such as this increases the likelihood of her developing postnatal depression. You can contact Victim Support and Women's Aid for support and counselling – see Useful Addresses.

Sexual abuse past or present

Having a baby can bring back the horrific memories of sexual abuse the mother may have suffered in the past. Like domestic violence, it can often raise a number of concerns in her mind. If the sexual abuse is still happening, she may be wondering how to prevent the baby witnessing her abuse, or whether she can protect the baby from her abuser. If she was abused in the past, she may worry that she may abuse the baby herself. Evidence shows, however, that this is unlikely. These situations can put a new mother under a great deal of strain, which could lead to postnatal depression. You can contact the Rape & Sexual Abuse Support Centre for support and counselling – see Useful Addresses.

These are all negative situations. It would be unusual for someone, say, to lose their partner and not feel sad. Sadness is a normal reaction to a negative life event. Happiness is a normal reaction to a positive life event.

Not every mother who experiences any or some of the above will experience postnatal depression. It is very difficult to predict just who will be affected. For you, having a baby at this time may have been the straw that broke the camel's back.

You may have identified the potential cause, or causes, of your feelings from this list. At the very least it may have got you thinking about yourself, your past experiences, and your present circumstances. Let's start thinking about your future.

3
Getting well

Early detection of postnatal depression is important in ensuring a quick recovery. The first and most important step on the road to recovery is that you, your partner and your family accept that this is temporary and that given time you will recover. The sooner you get support, the sooner you will recover.

Who can help me?

There are many people who can help you. They do not necessarily need to be trained experts, and they certainly do not need to have experienced postnatal depression to be able to support you. They do have one thing in common, though: they all care about you and want you to be well again. They may include the following:

- A range of NHS health professionals, such as your midwife, health visitor, GP, counsellors, psychotherapists and community psychiatric nurses.
- A range of independent practitioners, such as counsellors, psychotherapists and complementary therapists.
- Volunteers from organizations such as Home-Start and the Association of Postnatal Illness.
- Your partner and members of your family, such as your mum, your dad, your grandma and/or your sister.
- Friends, both those you have known for years and those you have become closer to since you have been pregnant or had your baby, because they have a young family too.
- Last but not least, and certainly most importantly, yourself.

You are the single most influential person in getting you well. Whatever happens, wherever you are, whoever you are with, you are always with you. You can be your own first port of call when it comes to support. This may sound a little strange at the moment, it may even sound like too much for you to cope with, but all will become clear in Chapter 4.

You may feel that you have no one – no partner, family or friends – to support you and that the only people who care for you are those that are paid to. But for now, do try to look on the bright side; you do have the health professionals, the independent practitioners, the volunteers and yourself to get you through this difficult time. How your partner, family and friends can help you is specifically talked about in Chapter 6. If you can get them to read any of this book, I would strongly encourage them to read this chapter and Chapter 6.

This chapter outlines the usual care offered to a woman suffering from postnatal depression, and the range of treatment options available through the NHS, together with additional sources of treatment such as complementary therapies and volunteer organizations.

The usual care offered by the NHS

As I have just encouraged you to get your partner, your family and/ or your friends to read this chapter, I will assume that the reader of this section could be any one of these people, including the woman who is postnatally depressed.

Basically, the usual care offered to a woman by the NHS will depend upon the severity of her postnatal depression.

To help find out if a woman is feeling depressed, and just how depressed, it is likely that her health visitor will ask her to fill in the Edinburgh Postnatal Depression Scale about six weeks after the birth. This is the questionnaire I mentioned in Chapter 1. As I said before, the health visitor will be using her clinical judgement (her years of training and experience) in combination with this questionnaire. A score of 12 or more (out of 30) on the questionnaire would tell her that a woman is vulnerable to developing the illness of postnatal depression.

If a woman scores 12 or more, her health visitor will probably offer to come and see her at home to talk about how she is feeling. Many health visitors call these 'listening visits', as their main aim is to listen to the woman talk about how she is feeling. They may also make suggestions about ways of coping with things that are bothering her, and about support groups that she could go along to.

Her health visitor may also recommend that she go and see her GP to talk about how she is feeling. The GP will be able to offer her forms of treatment that her health visitor cannot, including referral to counsellors, psychotherapists or community psychiatric nurses, and perhaps antidepressant medication.

A woman may not need to see a psychiatrist, but do not worry if her GP recommends that she does and refers her to one. Her GP will refer her to a psychiatrist only if it is necessary. Psychiatrists who work in this field are known as 'perinatal' psychiatrists and are sometimes attached to the department of liaison psychiatry in your local hospital. Quite often these days, perinatal psychiatrists have teams of specialist community psychiatric nurses who can offer home visits in between hospital appointments.

It is important to remember that all of these health professionals are trained to help the postnatally depressed mother; they do not want to lock her up, and they do not want to take her baby away from her. They want to help her to be well again as soon as possible. In addition, the usual care offered to a woman by the NHS will depend upon her response to the treatment offered and received. For example, one woman may find that talking to her health visitor on a regular basis in her own home may be enough to help her start to feel well. Another woman with a similar severity of postnatal depression may receive that same support but notice no real improvement in her illness; she may then also be offered antidepressant medication by her GP, an appointment with a psychiatrist, and a community psychiatric nurse to talk to on a regular basis in her own home, to help her start to feel well.

About one in four women suffering from postnatal depression develop more severe symptoms such as feeling suicidal, and naturally need more specialized, hospital-based care. In-patient care is rare unless a woman has severe depression. In your local area there will be specialist mother-and-baby facilities so that mothers needing this kind of help do not have to be separated from their babies while they are helped to recover in hospital.

Whatever treatment a woman receives, be it home visits from her health visitor or a stay in her local mother-and-baby unit, this will form part of an overall strategy of treatment. Support and practical help involving partners, family and friends is invaluable throughout this time. She will need a lot of support around her both during her hospital stay and when she goes home.

Throughout this book I have encouraged the woman who has, or thinks she has, postnatal depression, to talk to her midwife, health visitor or GP as soon as she can. It is important for her to speak to whichever one of them she can be honest with, as they are trained to help her. If she does not feel she can cope with explaining how she feels to a health professional on her own, she needs someone she trusts to be with her. As her partner, mum or friend, you could ask her midwife, health visitor or GP to come and see you both at home if she prefers. Please support her if she asks you to do this with her, or even offer to organize it for her.

Unfortunately, we do not live in a perfect world, and health professionals are just as capable of making mistakes and being stressed as the rest of us. If a woman with possible postnatal depression tells a health professional how she is feeling but receives no help, or not the help she feels she wants, she will need courage to raise the matter with them again or to speak to another health professional, as it is important that they take her seriously and that she is offered the help she needs. You as her partner, mum or friend, someone she trusts, can help to give her the courage to do that. Please, please do.

The usual treatments offered by the NHS

There are a number of treatments available to treat postnatal depression, and these treatments can be combined. The methods most widely offered and found to be helpful are talking therapies such as counselling and psychotherapy, and medication in the form of antidepressants. For some women a combination of antidepressants and counselling results in an enhanced rate of recovery. Having spoken to your doctor you can decide, together, whether receiving both treatments might help you to recover more quickly.

There are drawbacks to both forms of treatment. For example:

- Antidepressants can take between two and four weeks before they reach sufficient levels in your body to have any positive impact on your depression.
- You may experience unpleasant side effects that are unacceptable, such as increased appetite, weight gain and drowsiness.
- An appointment to see a counsellor or therapist may involve a long waiting list.
- You may not be able to establish a good relationship with the counsellor or therapist.

At the beginning of my career I was very opposed to the treatment of depression by medication; I felt that therapy was the answer. Taking tablets does not identify the cause of the depression, it simply masks the symptoms. As soon as a person stops taking the medication, if they have not made changes to the aspects of their life that make them unhappy and potentially cause the depression, then the depression may return. My view was that it is not a long-term cure but a short-term cover-up.

However, counselling and therapy requires a person to have some energy and be able to think fairly clearly about themselves and their life. Obviously this is not possible when someone is suffering from a severe depressive illness. Therefore, women with severe postnatal depression, if they were only offered therapy, would not benefit from it as much and probably not recover as quickly as women with mild to moderate postnatal depression. This quite rapidly struck me as being unfair and so I began to question my beliefs and myself.

Surely it would be better for a woman to have antidepressant medication to help lift her mood so that she can then take full part in any therapy or counselling she is offered? I think so. Witnessing many women battling with postnatal depression over the years has taught me this.

I now firmly believe that there is a place for any treatment that a woman perceives helps her, whether that be medication, therapy, reflexology, a walk to the shops, digging the garden, a soak in the bath, a foot rub, a cup of tea and a gossip with a friend, or throwing darts at a poster of a celebrity got-it-all actress/model/wife/mother/ fashion icon. Basically, if it makes you happy, it can't be that bad.

Therapy

Confiding in someone who is neither related to you nor a close friend may seem awkward at first but it does have some advantages. In particular, you may feel able to be more honest with the counsellor, as they will not take offence if you don't take their advice. In counselling, the opportunity to talk about your troubles to a sympathetic, understanding, uncritical ear can provide a great sense of relief and release.

Professional counselling can be a great help if you are depressed. Many GP practices in the UK now have access to a counselling or psychotherapy service. Your doctor may recommend you to a trained professional, which may be your midwife or your health visitor, who may offer to come and see you at home to talk through your difficulties with you. This may or may not be in addition to your health visitor offering you 'listening visits'.

If, however, your local GP practice does not offer this access to counselling or psychotherapy, or if the waiting time for an appointment is too long for you, you might consider seeking help from a private practitioner. If you have a private health care policy, check if you are covered for any mental health support, although unfortunately on most policies this is unlikely. If you decide to seek a counsellor or therapist for yourself then it is worth contacting the British Association for Counselling and Psychotherapy and/or the British Association for Behavioural and Cognitive Psychotherapies. They can provide you with information about therapists in your local area – see Useful Addresses for their contact details.

What types of therapy are available?

There are as many 'styles' of therapy as there are therapists. Your therapist will give you detailed information about the type he or she uses, but the usual kinds of therapy are:

- *Behaviour therapy*: this seeks to change your behaviour rather than your underlying personality, and encourages new 'coping' techniques.
- *Cognitive behavioural therapy*: in addition to seeking to change your behaviour, this type of therapy seeks to change negative thinking patterns.
- *Interpersonal psychotherapy*: this focuses on interpersonal relationships and coping with conflicts in relationships.
- *Psychodynamic therapy*: this focuses on underlying drives and desires that determine behaviour.

Think carefully about what type of therapy might suit you, taking into consideration what you think may be causing or contributing to your depression, and, for example, a therapy that is sensitive to your culture.

Therapy must have a cultural context that is meaningful. For example, research has shown that, in general, Asian women are traditionally brought up to have an indirect approach to expressing their needs and feelings, so for them something like assertiveness training would be of little or no use. In China, women tend to express their depression through physical symptoms such as headaches, backaches and so on, and not through psychological symptoms. Interpersonal therapy, with its focus on relationships, seems to be an effective type of treatment for them. This may be because their personal relationships are extremely important and can be the focal point of their self-definition – although this also tends to be true for many women. So if you are living in a society that is not of your own culture, when seeking a therapist try to find one whose training has made them culturally sensitive.

For mild to moderate depression, psychotherapy can be very beneficial. One form of psychotherapy, cognitive behavioural therapy (CBT), has been shown to be as effective as antidepressants. CBT involves looking at how you think about things, confronting negative thoughts and focusing your attention on positive thoughts and actions.

I have included a selection of these techniques in Chapter 4. If you would like to know more about CBT in general I would recommend you read Paul Gilbert's book, *Overcoming Depression: A Self-help Guide using Cognitive Behavioural Techniques*. Details of this and other books can be found in Further Reading.

How long will therapy take?

Therapy for depression can show results quickly, usually in a matter of weeks. You may choose to have a brief period of therapy to help you get through your postnatal depression and learn skills for coping with your life as a mum, or you could stay in therapy for a longer period of time (months as opposed to weeks) as a means of continuing your personal growth.

You might feel that a brief therapy is preferable to you as a mother, as you may feel that time is of the essence. The best brief therapy for depression is action-oriented. Basically, you need to know two things in order for you to start to recover:

• What is making you unhappy?
• What can you do about it?

When the therapy includes a clear action plan, such as keeping a feelings diary (as described in Chapter 4), the success rate of brief therapy with depression can go up to as much as 80 to 90 per cent.

How does therapy work?

Psychotherapy offers you the opportunity to identify the factors that contribute to your depression and helps you learn how to deal effectively with the psychological, behavioural, interpersonal and situational causes of it. Therapists work with depressed individuals to:

- Identify negative situations in their life that contribute to their depression, and help them understand which aspects of those problems they may be able to change. They can help depressed patients identify hopes for the future.
- Identify negative thinking patterns that contribute to feelings of hopelessness and helplessness that accompany depression. For instance, depressed people may tend to think of circumstances as extremes, such as things 'always going wrong' or 'never working out right'. They may also take events personally. A therapist can help nurture a more positive outlook on life.
- Explore other thoughts and behaviours that contribute to depression. For example, they may help a person to understand and change the way they talk, or don't talk, to others, if that is a cause of their depression.
- Help people get a sense of control and pleasure in life, encouraging them to see what choices they have and gradually to take up enjoyable activities.

How can I get the most from therapy?

All therapy is a two-way process. It works best when patients and their therapists talk honestly and openly. The outcome of psychotherapy is improved when both parties agree early on about what the major problems are and how psychotherapy can help.

You both have responsibilities in establishing and maintaining a good working relationship. Be clear with your therapist about any hopes and fears you may have about therapy. Therapy will work better and more quickly when you attend all the appointments and give some thought to what you have discussed between each session.

How can I tell if therapy is helping?

After two or three sessions, if you feel the experience is truly a joint effort and that you enjoy a good relationship with your therapist, you are making progress. Speak to your therapist if you don't feel

31

positive about it, or if you find yourself thinking about stopping your therapy.

It is usual to feel a wide range of emotions during therapy. You may have some uncomfortable feelings while having therapy, as a result of discussing painful and concerning experiences. Be reassured, though, that this is positive – it is a sign that you are starting to explore your own thoughts and behaviours for yourself. Therapy isn't necessarily the easy option.

Medication

As discussed in Chapter 2, the exact cause of depression is not known. Evidence indicates that it is caused by a chemical imbalance in the brain, which could be a result of your genetic predisposition, or triggered by events in your life. This chemical imbalance indicates that there aren't enough chemical messengers (neurotransmitters) in the brain. These neurotransmitters carry messages (nerve impulses) from one nerve cell to another. Sometimes there aren't enough of these messengers, and certain messages don't get carried to some areas of the brain. Two primary messengers, called serotonin and norepinephrine, are responsible for how you feel.

More than 20 medicines treat depression and these medicines are called antidepressants. They help to increase the number of these chemical messengers, serotonin and norepinephrine. There are two main kinds of antidepressants: the tricyclic antidepressants (TCAs) and the selective serotonin reuptake inhibitors (SSRIs).

How will my GP or psychiatrist pick an antidepressant for me?

Your GP or psychiatrist will take a number of things into account when choosing an antidepressant medicine for you. They will consider, for example:

- Which medicine will help you, as quickly as possible, with the most negative and disabling symptoms of your depression.
- If you are breastfeeding. The medication may have an effect on you and your breastfed baby.
- Which is the best medicine for you. That is, the one that gives you the fewest and least serious side effects.

- If you have had depression before. If you took an antidepressant previously and it helped, your doctor may prescribe it again.
- If any of your close relatives – parents, brothers, sisters – have had depression. If they have taken a certain antidepressant and it worked well for them, that medicine might be good for you too.
- Any existing physical health problems and the medication you take for them. There may be possible negative interactions between other medicines and antidepressants.
- How often you want to take the antidepressant. The less often you need to take the tablets, the less likely you are to forget and miss a dose; and the sooner you are likely to start to feel well again.

Are there cultural differences in the prescription of antidepressants?

It is important that whoever prescribes your medication understands the biological differences between the ethnic groups relevant to your case, and has experience in prescribing drugs for them. People from different ethnic backgrounds metabolize drugs differently. The dosage may need to be quite different.

Do antidepressants cause side effects?

Yes. All antidepressants have some side effects that will affect some people. Like most medications, this does not necessarily mean that *you* will actually experience them.

What are some of the common side effects?

The side effects vary with different medicines. In general, SSRIs have fewer side effects than most TCAs, and may for this reason be preferable in postnatal depression.

Some of the possible side effects of TCAs include the following: blurred vision, increased sleepiness, muscle tremors, feeling of weakness, weight gain, increased heart rate, and dizziness when standing up. Some of these may be particularly serious for you as the mother of a young baby. In addition, the information leaflet inside the packet will recommend that you do not drive or operate machines while taking the drug, because it may affect your reflexes and your attention span. Obviously a restriction on driving might also make parenting difficult.

SSRIs may cause the following side effects: nausea, muscle tremors, sexual dysfunction (inability to ejaculate or to have an orgasm), increased sleepiness, decreased sleepiness, and increased anxiety. Again, some of these may be unacceptable for you as the mother of a young baby.

What if the side effects don't go away?

Talk to whoever prescribed you the medication. He or she may change your dosage or you might try another medicine to relieve the side effects.

Can I breastfeed if I am taking antidepressants?

Medication, as with food and drink, affects breast milk. It is well known that alcohol, for instance, can pass in large amounts quite quickly from mother to child via breast milk. Antidepressants can pass from mother to child through breast milk, but the balance of risks and benefits to the mother in taking antidepressants must be considered. Many doctors feel that the benefits of a contented mother breastfeeding and bonding with her baby, while on antidepressant medication, outweigh the possible risks of a small amount of the antidepressant reaching the child. Some mothers do, however, prefer to bottle-feed while taking antidepressants.

Could antidepressants affect my child in later life?

Several studies have been carried out to see whether antidepressants affect how the brain works in children as they mature. Reassuringly, at the time of writing, no delayed effects on behaviour have been found in children exposed to antidepressants through breast milk.

Are antidepressants tranquillizers?

No. These tablets are not tranquillizers.

Can I get addicted to antidepressants?

There is currently no conclusive evidence that antidepressants are chemically addictive. However, some people feel that they are reliant upon them; they become a crutch to get them through the day. This is why combining antidepressant medication with some form of therapy or counselling is important. Therapy encourages you to begin to gather strength and confidence within yourself that overtakes any artificially created buoyancy supplied by antidepressants.

When finishing a course of antidepressants it is important to come off them gradually, cutting down the dose over a period of time. Your GP or psychiatrist who prescribed the medication will advise on this. Stopping an antidepressant suddenly can lead to a reoccurrence of the depression.

How will I know if my antidepressant is working?

Remember that antidepressants take two or more weeks before they work – so don't give up just because you don't feel any better immediately. Basically, you will know that your antidepressant is working when you begin to feel well: if you start sleeping better, feel like you want to take more care of yourself (such as looking after your appearance and eating regularly), have more energy, and/or feel an increased desire to live and take part in life. Your family and friends will also notice these changes. Your GP or psychiatrist will check your progress by asking you about these things.

How long will I take the antidepressant for?

If this is the first time you have been treated for depression, you will probably continue taking the medicine for about six months after you first feel an improvement in your symptoms. If you have had depression before, you might expect to take the medicine for at least a year after you begin to feel well. It is important to continue to take the antidepressant after your depression has lifted, to prevent it returning. Six to twelve months might seem like a very long time, but if it means that you then stay well, it will obviously be worth it. Always bear in mind that depression is an illness, and give yourself time to recover.

Additional sources of treatment

There is a wide range of independent practitioners offering additional help, including counsellors, psychotherapists and complementary therapists, and volunteers from organizations such as Home-Start and the Association of Postnatal Illness. As discussed above, whether they are independent or NHS-employed, counsellors and psychotherapists will help you in the same way – the only difference is in what it will cost you. We now focus on complementary therapies and volunteer organizations.

Complementary therapies

Complementary therapies, such as reflexology and aromatherapy, have been found to help women suffering from postnatal depression. As their name suggests, these therapies are most effective when used to complement other treatments: the majority of complementary therapists do not advise that their treatments be used as an alternative to those offered by the NHS. You can try these therapies alongside the treatment recommended by your doctor, and many women have found that a combination of treatments really helps them.

There are many therapies available, including:

- *Aromatherapy*: said to be one of the oldest forms of natural healing. It uses powerful plant essences (essential oils) and massage to help stimulate the body's healing processes and immune systems. When carried out by a properly qualified therapist aromatherapy can be an effective and beneficial treatment of natural healthcare, with few if any side effects.
- *Acupuncture*: can relieve symptoms of some physical and psychological conditions and may encourage the patient's body to heal and repair itself, if it is able to do so. It is said to work by stimulating the nerves in skin and muscle, and can produce a variety of effects. It has been found to increase the body's release of natural painkillers – endorphin and serotonin – in the pain pathways of both the spinal cord and the brain. This modifies the way pain signals are received. It can not only reduce pain but is said to improve an individual's sense of well-being.
- *Herbal remedies*: many of these exist but one in particular is relevant for depression, St John's Wort. However, it has been shown to be beneficial for only mild depression. Despite it having few known side effects, certain precautions should be taken when trying this remedy, such as avoiding direct sunlight, strong cheese and red wine, and not taking the herb Ephedra. It is also not known how or if St John's Wort interacts with other medication. You must tell your GP if you are taking this herbal remedy, so they can take this into consideration when prescribing for other ailments.
- *Reflexology*: thought to date back 3,000 years, to the ancient Egyptians. It is based on the principle that the body is represented in the feet and it was found that if the feet were worked on, this improved health physically and emotionally. By massaging the reflex points on the feet or hands, subtle energy within the body is stimulated via the nervous system. Reflexology can help many ailments, as it helps to balance all the systems of the body to work and support each other.

- *Homeopathy*: said to have no harmful side effects; a special preparation process called potentization refines the medicines to remove any toxic effects. It is considered so safe that it is suitable for taking during pregnancy, although obviously special care must be taken with any medication taken while you are pregnant. The tablets or solutions work by stimulating the body's own natural defence mechanism.

Bear in mind that complementary therapies are often only available privately, and cost may be a consideration for you. Contact individual therapists directly to find out how much each session costs.

You need to be confident that the person offering the therapy is properly trained. The best way to ensure this is to contact the regulatory body for the specific therapy. Often there is a national register provided by the regulatory body and only fully qualified therapists can be listed on the register. It is worth contacting the Institute for Complementary Medicine and/or, more specifically, the British Reflexology Association or the British Acupuncture Council, who can provide you with information about therapists in your local area. These organizations are listed in Useful Addresses.

Baby massage

You may also like to learn how to massage your child. Infant or baby massage has been found to benefit both mother and baby as individuals, and it may enhance the bond between you. Many midwives and health visitors are becoming trained in infant or baby massage, and there may be a group that meets near you. Ask your GP, midwife or health visitor about this, or contact the Guild of Infant and Child Massage and/or the International Association of Infant Massage and ask for details of their qualified professional members. Contact details for these organizations are listed in Useful Addresses.

Volunteer organizations

There are a number of organizations run by volunteers who work together to help mothers with postnatal depression and their partners and families. In many cases, the people who work for these charities (as they tend to be) have experienced postnatal depression them-selves. Again, they all have one thing in common, and that is that they care about you and want you to be well again. Some organizations have groups that meet locally, so you can go along and gain support both from the volunteers and other women who are suffering or have recovered from postnatal depression. These include MAMA (Meet A Mum Association) and Depression Alliance.

Some organizations have telephone helplines, numbers you can call whenever you are feeling down and want to talk to someone who will offer you sympathy and understanding. These days they often also offer email contact, in case you would prefer not to speak to someone directly. All those listed in Useful Addresses have a website where you can gather useful information. See, for instance, the Samaritans, CRY-SIS, Parentline Plus, the Association for Postnatal Illness.

One charity, Home-Start, offers to match a volunteer in your area to you and your family, to come and see you in your home and provide you with practical and emotional support. Some Home-Start areas also offer support groups for all local mothers of young children, not necessarily just for those with postnatal depression.

All these organizations and more are listed in Useful Addresses, under the headings 'Depression', 'Parenting and family life' and 'Postnatal depression'.

4

How you can help yourself to get well

This chapter outlines how you can help yourself to get well and the usual pattern of recovery you can expect to experience.

There are many ways you can help yourself to feel well again. It is undeniably true that whatever happens, wherever you are, whoever you are with, you are always with you. You are always available to support yourself through anything. That means that you are the single most influential person in getting you well.

As I said earlier, if you are currently feeling depressed, the thought of being your own first port of call may just be too much for you to cope with at the moment. You probably feel that right now you don't have the energy to help get yourself through this illness. But you must try and believe that this will change. As you start to feel better it will become easier for you to manage this.

There are a number of ways you can help yourself through postnatal depression, alongside the treatments offered by and as alternatives to the NHS. These can all be combined to enhance your recovery.

Later in this chapter I will describe some practical ideas you can try to help yourself feel better. First, it is important that you understand the importance of trying to accept that your life is different now; you need to be as realistic as possible about your life, and accept how you feel at the moment, that is, postnatally depressed. Once you have thought about and accepted these things you will be better prepared and more motivated to try out the ideas that follow.

Life is different now

Try to accept that life has changed

Capabilities differ not just between people but also within people. At different times in our lives we feel stronger and more capable than at other times. In different situations we may feel more or less able to cope, and this may be due to our perception of our own ability in that situation. That is, one person may consider she is good at maths and

39

so finds budgeting the household finances easy; however, that same woman may also think she is a bad cook and so the thought of having to nourish a baby to help it grow up into a fit and healthy child fills her with a cold dread.

When we are in new situations, generally, we try not to put ourselves under too much pressure. Having a new baby is a new situation. It differs from most others, however, in that babies do not allow you to have breaks, rarely have a routine and are dependent upon you (and your partner). So although you may not be putting yourself under pressure, at least one little bundle may be.

In addition, you may feel pressure from others and society in general to be capable all the time, to enjoy your baby all the time, to anticipate your baby's needs all the time, and to want to be with your baby all the time. If you don't feel this way, all the time, you may start putting pressure on yourself to at least appear to the outside world that you do. Obviously this is not helpful and is not realistic.

Try to be realistic in your expectations

Most women, before they get pregnant and/or while they are pregnant, think about how life will be when the baby arrives. These thoughts might include wondering what the baby will look like, hoping that they won't cry too much, hoping that she will make a good mother, and that her partner will be a good father.

As outlined in Chapter 2, if a woman's expectations of life as a mother are realistic, then she will be less likely to be depressed postnatally. If, however, her ideas of life with a young baby and how she will cope with it verge on fantasy or perfection then she will be more at risk of feeling let down by the reality of motherhood.

Aspiring to perfection is not a bad thing in itself. We all do it. The desire to be the best mother we can possibly be is a natural drive to try and ensure that we take the best care we can of our child. This maximizes the chances of our offspring surviving to adulthood to produce offspring of their own. It's nature. The important thing to note here is that aspiring to be perfect is very different from expecting to be perfect. As long as we accept that none of us is perfect, and nor are we as individuals ever likely to achieve perfection, there is not a problem.

When I am working with groups of pregnant women, we often talk about their expectations of motherhood. It is useful, as I said earlier, to think about how life will be, as this helps us prepare for the challenges ahead. So just in case they haven't thought about it much, I ask them to write a job description for the post of 'mother'. I encourage them to think about what they would be doing on a typical day. The job description has to include the following:

- hours of duty
- standard and comfort of working environment
- necessary prior experience of this role or similar roles in the past
- equipment it will be necessary to operate
- access to transport
- pay
- holiday entitlements
- cover for holiday
- the roles of other team members.

Needless to say, when they start to think about it in these terms, some women get a bit of a shock. You might be one of those women. The simple reality of motherhood is that it isn't glamorous, it isn't well paid, it is often dreadfully repetitive, it is often carried out on your own, and it can be very stressful. Of course it does have wonderful heart-stopping, stomach-flipping, face-splitting ecstatic times too. So, it is important to have a balanced image of motherhood, and that includes both negative and positive aspects.

Try to accept how you feel
You will have changed after having your baby. You may think you have changed too much, or too little. You may think you haven't changed in the way that you ought to have. Perhaps you don't like the person you seem to have changed into. You may feel that this change has happened without you having any control over it.

If that is the case and you don't like how you have changed, you may well now be wondering whether you will ever regain control over yourself sufficiently to change to how you want to be. Try not to worry about that at the moment; it is good that you are thinking about how you feel. Slowly but surely, as you recover, you will begin to feel that you want to have control over your life and feel more like the person you want to be.

The best thing you can do right now is to accept that you feel the way you do. Don't be frightened of thinking about how you feel, and what makes you feel like that. Once you start to think about what might be causing your depression then you, with the help of others, can start to change those depressing feelings into ones that you would like to be feeling.

When we are feeling unsure of ourselves it is usual to look around us and compare ourselves to others in a similar situation to ourselves, or so we think. This gives us some information as to how we are doing in the 'being a good mother' stakes. However, as each of us is different, comparing ourselves with others is of only limited use, especially as when we are depressed we tend to be much harsher on ourselves than on others.

We also often have no information to go on beyond the surface appearance of other people, and so we cannot compare and contrast accurately. So if you find yourself coming off second-best in those irresistible moments of 'look at her, she looks so organized and her baby looks really happy and content', remember that it may simply be that she is better at hiding her postnatal depression than you. Even if she is convincingly happy, it may be that she has been wearing the mask that says all is well in her life for so long now that she can't remember how to take it off.

Or perhaps she really is happy. Really happy. This may, in fact it probably will, make you feel envious. Envy is a very negative emotion. Although it is directed outwards at others, it often leaves a scar inside, and a residual taste of guilt for wishing someone else ill. Depression is often maintained by negative thinking. So try to stop asking, 'why me?' and actually start doing something about accepting yourself, and all other mothers, as a 'good enough mother'.

Practical ideas

The following ideas will take energy and effort to do. Don't feel that you should get on with any or all of them straight away. Just reading about these ideas and thinking about what you might be able to do later is good enough for now. It counts as actually doing something.

What would be useful, while reading through these ideas, is to start to plan how you could try to do them. Then when you feel ready to put those plans into action, the energy you have at that point in the future will be being better spent doing what you have already given some thought to. See how you feel.

The following topics cover those areas of everyday life that women with postnatal depression, in my experience, have valued getting practical ideas about. Many of these ideas have their basis in cognitive behavioural therapy. You may feel that some of them are more relevant to you than others. Just read through and see what you think. If they don't click with you at the moment, it may be that when you are further along the road to recovery they will appeal to you more. For now, it will be useful for you just to be aware of what you could try to do.

These suggestions are drawn from an information pack called *Helping New Mothers to Help Themselves* (© Potent) that I wrote for health professionals, such as health visitors and midwives, who work with women who have postnatal depression. Details of how to obtain the complete pack can be found in Further Reading.

Successfully solving everyday problems

Quite simply the most effective way to solve problems successfully is to learn to *plan* solving them thoroughly. It is a good way of building up your confidence. You may already know how useful this method of problem-solving is, and if so this section will act as a reminder to help you to continue planning your solutions thoroughly.

Successful problem-solving involves six stages:

1 Identifying exactly what the problem is.
2 Thinking about the ways you could try to solve that problem.
3 Deciding which is the best way for you to try and solve that problem.
4 Attempting to solve that problem in that way.
5 Assessing whether that action did solve that problem.
6 Praising yourself for applying your solution to the problem.

This may seem like a lot of work as it is written down here, but it is something that all of us do, at least in part, on a daily basis. The first five stages are what most of us do all the time in our heads. We realize there is a problem, we wonder what to do, we work out what we can do, we do it, and then we check if it worked. What we are all pretty bad at is the last stage – thinking to ourselves that we did a good job, or even if we didn't solve the problem, identifying which bits we did do well. We should try to remember what made that success happen and think about how we can apply the success-producing elements to other problems that will occur in our lives.

If you can learn to praise your efforts, not just the results of your efforts, you will be well on the road to successful problem-solving. When something doesn't work out as well as you had hoped, you will feel more able to have another go. It will make it more likely that you will succeed second time around. In fact it will make you more likely to succeed full stop.

It is often said that we learn more from our mistakes than from our successes. We all make mistakes. Anyone who says they never make mistakes is mistaken.

What will help your attempts to solve problems to be successful is breaking down one seemingly huge problem into smaller parts. For example, you have postnatal depression and you want to be well again. Many small aspects of your life need to change to solve this problem and help you recover. It simply is not possible to solve this problem in one plan with the six stages shown above.

Problem-solving and postnatal depression

How do you eat an elephant? The answer is, of course, one mouthful at a time.

You cannot solve the problem of having postnatal depression and wanting to be well again in one fell swoop. It is an elephant. You need to start with something smaller and more achievable. That way you are setting yourself up to feel better about yourself, as your plan will be more likely to work when you put it in to practice.

Let's take the example of a smaller problem to be solved: 'you would like more time for yourself'. Using the above six stages as a guide, we can plan how to solve this problem. I will fill it in as if it were my own problem. Planning how to solve the problem consists of the first four stages, as follows.

1 *Identify exactly what the problem is.*
I would like more time for myself.

2 *Think about the ways you could try to solve that problem. If possible, think of at least three, to give you some choices.*
- I could ask my partner/mother/friend to have the baby while I put my feet up for half an hour.
- I could find out if I can put my baby in the crèche at the leisure centre while I have a swim.

- I could try to relax while the baby is sleeping in the daytime, instead of tidying up and doing the ironing.

3 *Decide which is the best way for you to try to solve that problem. Think about the practicalities of each choice; compare them with each other and consider your own ability to actually carry out the solutions you have come up with.*

The third is possibly the most realistic one as it doesn't involve me asking anybody else for help. I just have to be firm with myself and ignore the ironing. I might try the first one at some time in the future if this goes well – but I won't do it now because I will have to ask others to help me, and the baby has to get used to being away from me. I could offer to have my friend's baby another time in exchange and I won't have to pay her.

4 *Attempt to solve that problem in that way. Think about what you will physically need to do, in what order, to give yourself the best chance of successfully solving this problem.*

To try and relax while the baby is sleeping in the daytime I need to put the ironing pile somewhere I can't see it from the sofa, and make sure the vacuum cleaner is out of sight too. I could have a magazine ready and/or maybe a video of a programme I want to watch from the other night. I could even have filled the kettle and put the tea bag in the cup. That way I can make the best use of the time I get when she does finally go to sleep.

Once you have planned how to solve a problem, you then have to try out your plan. The final two stages enable you to evaluate what went well, what you could have done differently, and how well you did at various stages.

5 *Assess whether that action did solve that problem. Decide how you will know the problem is solved; you can decide this for yourself and/or ask others what they think.*

When she eventually went to sleep I had 25 minutes to put my feet up and have a cup of tea. But instead of watching my video I fell asleep! At least I was relaxed . . .

6 *Praise yourself for applying the solution to the problem. Think about how you expected it to go – did you think it would be more or*

less difficult than it actually was? You know that simply doing a plan and putting it into action is something to feel proud of on its own. How will you reward yourself?

I tried to anticipate all the possible distractions, like hiding the ironing, which really did help me to relax – it shows how well I know myself and that is good! I will reward myself by doing this again tomorrow or the next day.

You will be more successful in solving everyday problems more quickly if you write down your thoughts. At the end of this chapter are some guide sheets that you can fill in. Try to plan, and then evaluate, how to solve some of your problems successfully – once you have broken them down into smaller, easier-to-swallow sections, that is.

Thinking positively about yourself and your life

We are affected on a daily basis by the things we experience in our lives. Whether we are usually a pessimist or an optimist, having an illness like depression makes us all become more pessimistic. Like pessimists, we begin to expect things to go wrong. In fact, when we are depressed we actually tend to look for things that have gone wrong to prove to ourselves that we were right to expect that they would. How depressing!

So, how you feel directly affects what you think. Likewise, what you think affects how you feel. Fortunately, this is true for both good experiences and bad. When something happens to make you feel happy, you are more optimistic afterwards.

We all know that we have little control over what happens to us in our lives on a daily basis; for example, babies don't sleep when we want them to. We are unlikely to be able to control how we *feel* about that situation either, but what we can do much more easily is control what we *think* about it. You *can* make a difference to yourself and your life. What you think could make all the difference in the world to how you feel.

The reason why this particular practical idea is so useful and effective is because you can gain instant control over what you think. Pretty much as soon as you start to think positively, you will start to feel more positive too.

You reap what you sow – avoid negative thoughts

The best way to start is for you to think about the positive things you could say to yourself; statements that would help you feel better when things don't work out the way you had hoped they would. This overlaps with the sixth stage of successfully solving problems.

When something goes horribly wrong, you, like the rest of us, probably say to yourself, almost without thinking, something along the lines of (expletives deleted):

- Typical, that always happens to me.
- Just my luck, nothing ever goes right for me.
- Oh no, not again.
- Everything I do goes wrong.
- Why does it always happen to me?

You will notice that all these phrases are, first, negative, and second, very extreme. They suggest that we are consistently wrong, and would be stupid to think we would be anything but wrong. Although most of us do say these things to ourselves on a regular basis, it is not a good thing for anyone to do, particularly if we are depressed and more likely to believe that we are wrong and never will be right again.

If you find that once you start thinking negative thoughts they just don't stop coming, that is when you have to take control. *You* have to stop those vicious thoughts circling round *your* brain.

Get things in perspective

Ask yourself, how much will this 'disaster' matter to me in three months' time? How much of an effect will this, whatever has gone wrong, have on my life then? The honest answer is that the majority of things that happen in our everyday lives that make us angry, frustrated, irritated and/or plain exhausted, won't matter at all in three months' time. At a push they might still annoy us in three hours' time, but in all probability in three days' time we will struggle to remember what it was that got us so down. So when things go badly, try to put them into perspective – OK, it didn't go well, but is it the end of the world? Does it really mean that everything else in your life will always go wrong for you in the future?

No. This is what you have to try and do. You have to stand up to the depression and the hold that your illness has had, until now, on your thoughts and feelings. Ask yourself, and answer honestly, does everything really always go wrong for you? It can't possibly be that nothing has ever gone right for you. Remember that something must have gone right for you recently – you are reading this book and now you are thinking about how you can make yourself feel better.

Train yourself to be positive

We always find it difficult to praise ourselves when we have done something well; perhaps we fear the ridicule of others (and ourselves) that will go with appearing to be smug (sorry, I meant to say, appearing to be pleased).

Think about this: the phrase 'self-congratulatory' is generally used as a term of derision. And as part of you helping yourself get well, I want you to congratulate yourself at every available opportunity! Oh dear, as if it wasn't going to be difficult enough for you to feel better. In the light of the above, it is obviously important for you to know that I don't expect you to tell the world when you have done a good job. But I *do* want you to mention it to yourself. Lots. Again, and again, and again, until you believe that you have made something positive happen.

Focus on the positive things in your life. Think about them. Look for the good things that have happened to you. They may only be small things, but if they are good then focus on them. Notice and point out to yourself when things do work out better than you dared hope for. If you don't look for the positive things that happen in and around your life you will not see them. Remember what has made you feel happy; cherish that feeling with all the tenderness you can muster. And do it again, whatever it was that made you happy, if you can.

It will seem like impossibly hard work at first. There is no doubt at all about that. But you have to aim to take charge of your mind. You need to train yourself to think positively, train yourself to *be* positive, train yourself to look for the positives in the people around you, in the things that happen to you, and in the things that you do. You have to believe that there are positive things out there.

Right now it will feel like a complete leap of faith if you are at the bottom of your pit of despair. Please have faith in me. Trust me. Have the same faith in you that I have in you. You can do it. Thousands of women have done it, and you can too. I know it.

Positive statements

As I said, you can build up your confidence in general by praising yourself for your efforts, rather than only for the results of your actions. The statements below are examples of what some women say to themselves to build up their confidence, which they have mentioned to me over the years. They may ring a bell with you; if they don't, have a think about something you *could* say to yourself to cheer yourself up when things go wrong. Because they will go wrong, that's life.

- You can do this, you know.
- It will get better.
- It will be OK one day.
- I am doing the best I can.
- That's not bad for a first attempt.
- It may not be brilliant, but it will do for now.

Could you say any of these to yourself without sounding too trite? Put a mark next to those you think you could. Try to think of a couple of your own and write them down too. Remember that short and snappy phrases are easier to remember. And if they are easy to remember, you will be able to recall them more often, helping you feel better more quickly.

Build up slowly

When trying out these ideas for the first few times, go easy on yourself. Changing the focus of what you think towards dwelling on the positive may be possible for only limited periods of time. You are currently suffering from a serious illness, and the effort it will take to apply these suggestions will probably be more than you can manage for any length of time. The most helpful thing would be for you to build up your positive thinking gradually. Try it for, say, an hour a day for the first week and work your way up from there. If you find yourself getting exhausted, drop back a chunk of time and slowly build it up again. That way you will be becoming healthier with every passing week.

Alternatively, you may prefer to decide that 'from this point forward I will be positive'. It is entirely up to you; do what you consider will be the best way for you. You know yourself and your capabilities better than anyone. These are just suggestions that others have found useful, and I hope that you will too. Any positive change in your thinking is an improvement in your mental health and something you should feel good about having achieved. It is not easy when you feel down.

Remember that you don't have to do any of this on your own. Talk to someone you trust about what you are trying to do and ask them to support you. They could give it a go themselves – I think we could all do with being a bit more positive about ourselves.

Successfully seeking and accepting help

Most women are not very good at accepting offers of help. We would much prefer to cope on our own, and the result of this is that we often end up suffering on our own too. And if we are hung up about *accepting* offers of help, how often do you think we actually *ask* for help? Not often enough, of course.

It's not looking good so far, is it? And that is before you even include the fact that a woman with a young baby is probably the most likely to need help, but is the most likely to turn it down (let alone ask for it) lest she appear to the outside world that she is not coping and is, therefore, a bad mother.

Accepting offers of help

You will already have guessed that if someone offers you help, I would advise you to snatch his or her arm off. And if you feel that you don't know what to do or that you can't do something, you should ask someone you trust for help. None of us are idiots, we all know what we should do, but we are all desperately trying to avoid looking like idiots. The end result is that we find ourselves doing too much, feeling dreadful and eventually not being able to do very much at all.

What we must do is think about asking for and accepting help in a logical way. We have all had someone offering to help us with some minor task, and experienced the feeling of irritation that the reason they offered was because they thought you couldn't do it or complete it on your own, when you knew that you were doing just fine, thank you. Like I say, you are not an idiot. But you, like me, in that situation are being illogical.

You already know that the world doesn't revolve around you and how you feel; it follows that people offer you help because *they want* to help you. People want to help partly because it makes them feel good about themselves. They have done their good turn for the day. We all, as social animals, like to receive the praise of those around us. And what better way to receive praise than to offer help to someone else that they will say 'thank you' for? If you turn down offers of help you are not only making your own life hard, but also making the other person feel unwanted. Fact.

Asking for help

The same is true when you think logically about asking for help. Imagine how you would feel if you had to ask, say, your next-door neighbour if you could borrow £10, right now. How do you feel? Stop reading and look up from the page. Think about it for a moment. At first you probably thought, 'I couldn't do that! What would they think of me?' You would probably have then felt, even though you were only imagining it, embarrassed, awkward and ashamed: 'How awful.'

Now put yourself in the other person's position. Imagine that your next-door neighbour has just come round to see you, and asked to borrow £10. How would you feel? Again stop reading, look up from the page and think about those feelings for a moment. Notice that your reaction to my suggestion was probably not as immediate; you may not have felt anything particularly strongly at all. You probably thought, 'If I've got a tenner I can spare, she can have it.' You might have felt flattered that she felt she could come and ask you, have felt that you wanted to help if you possibly could. You may even have thought that you could lend her a fiver if that's all you could spare.

Notice the difference between these two perspectives. The person doing the asking usually feels all sorts of negative emotions and thinks unhelpful thoughts. The person being asked usually feels all sorts of positive emotions and thinks helpful thoughts. I don't know why two people in the same social interaction think and feel such opposite things, but they do.

What you should try to remember, and you have to believe me because I have just shown that it is true for you, and probably for everyone else reading this book, is that people generally like being asked to help. They also like to have their offers of help accepted. There is no need to cringe when you ask someone for help. There is no need to beat yourself up when you let someone help you. Ever.

Deciding what help you want from whom

As I have just shown you, help and support really is available to you. Any barrier you put between yourself and getting the help you want or need is of your own making. You can choose to climb over that barrier of being afraid to ask for or accept help in case people think you are incapable, at any time.

Now that you can remember to feel all right about asking for and accepting help by being logical, and remember how the other person usually feels better for having been asked to help or had their offer accepted, you need to think about who you would actually feel comfortable accepting it from. Help, be it practical or emotional, has to be acceptable to you, as well as available.

Who can you rely on?

I want you to think about who you feel you can rely on, people who have been there for you in the past, those you think might be there for you in the future. I don't just mean for the really big things, but for the little things as well. You may be able to come up instantly with five or six people, or you may struggle to think of two. Don't worry. What about friends you haven't seen recently or kept in touch with, but still feel you could talk to about almost anything? There may be someone you have met very recently, say at antenatal clinic, who you might be willing to ask for help. Think of as many people as you can.

Some women find it useful to think about what advice they would like someone to offer them in their situation. Then think about who would be most likely to say those things to you. Chances are that the person who would be able to offer the advice you would be most likely to take will be someone you feel you can trust. That person is an acceptable source of support.

I would like you to answer the questions in the following tables by writing, in the spaces provided, the names of all the people you can think of who might offer that type of help, and from whom it would be acceptable for you to receive that help. Remember to look further than your family and well-established friends; think about your new friends, your neighbours, and any health professionals you get on well with (midwife, health visitor, practice nurse).

Who could you ask for practical help? For example:

Doing the ironing.	
Cleaning the house.	
Looking after the baby for a few hours.	
Spending a wet afternoon with them.	
Going to the supermarket together.	

Who could you ask for advice? For example:

When you think the baby is ill.	
About starting the baby on solids.	
What benefits you are entitled to.	
Returning to work.	
How to handle your partner's requests for, or avoidance of, sex.	

Who could you ask for emotional support? For example:

Sharing your doubts and fears.	
Sharing your anger and resentment.	
Giving you encouragement and reassurance.	
Having a good cry with them.	
Laughing at yourself with them.	

Have a look at your answers. Are there any blank spaces? If there are, try not to worry about it, although it might be a good idea to think again. It may be that you truly don't have anyone that you could ask for that kind of help – or is it that you would really prefer not to have to ask anyone for that kind of help? There may be someone you might be able to ask for that kind of help in the future, for example someone you don't know well at the moment but hope to get to know better in time, another new mum perhaps.

Remember that the question asks you to think of who you *could* ask, not necessarily who you *have asked* in the past. Have another look at the questions bearing this in mind, and see if that helps you to fill the gaps. If it doesn't, don't worry about it for now. As you begin to recover, you will feel more confident and might be willing in the future to consider asking someone you wouldn't dream of asking at the moment. Stranger things have happened.

Be realistic about what you can expect from others

Does one person's name come up a lot for different sorts of support? For example, your mum, your partner, or your best friend? Try to be realistic about how many different things you could ask someone to help you with at any given time. Life is about give and take, and there has to be a balance. Could you really be there for them in that same way? Probably not, and that is not just because you have a serious illness at the moment.

You have to know your own limitations and not push yourself too hard; particularly now, but at any time in your life, you need to be aware of when you might be taking on more than is good for your mental health. Realizing that you are not invincible will help you to remember that other people have limitations too. If you can, think of other people you could ask for help that you would be equally happy accepting it from. Try to have an alternative person in mind in case they can't help. This overlaps with the second stage of planning how to successfully solve problems. It is always useful to have a range of options to choose from.

You may feel that you would like more help from certain people in your life. Perhaps you feel that those closest to you – your partner, your mother or your best friend – should know instinctively that you need help, what kind of help you need, and when you need it. But this is completely unrealistic. We can't say that we know telepathically when, where and how *they* need help at any given time, so why do we hope for it from them? It is just not possible. Help that you have received after deciding you needed it and then asked for is worth so much more to your health at this time. It is more valuable because you have put effort into it.

It is well known that the quickest and most effective way to change other people's behaviour is to change your own. By seeking and accepting help more often from those you feel you would like more support from, you are encouraging them to change too. Hopefully for the benefit of you all.

Put yourself higher up your priority list

As a new mum you may feel that you are in second place to the baby. The baby is your own, and everybody else's, priority. Before your needs or wants are met, those of the baby's have to be dealt with. So of course it is tempting to put yourself lower down the list of priorities; but make sure you are not bottom of the list. After all, who will mother your baby if you don't care for yourself and allow others to care for you? This involves caring for yourself physically and emotionally.

Your physical health influences your emotional health. So it would be a good idea to take some of the physical symptoms of postnatal depression described in Chapter 1 and work out ways that suit you of monitoring and improving them. Ask yourself the following questions, thinking about how you have looked after yourself in the last month. Be honest in your answers.

	Yes	No
Have you tried to get as much sleep as you can?		
Have you tried to eat healthy food?		
Have you tried not to drink coffee, tea, cola or alcohol?		
Have you tried to drink 4–8 glasses of water each day?		
Have you tried to get some exercise every day, for example a walk?		

If you got more ticks in the 'Yes' column than the 'No', that is great. Even if you said 'Yes' to all of them, you could probably, like most of us, do them more often. Think about how you might do each of these tasks more often. How could you try to achieve these simple things to help you stay fit and healthy, now and in the future? Please write your ideas for how you could do this in the space beneath each question. For example, instead of having a cup of tea, have a glass of water; or instead of doing the cleaning when the baby has a mid-morning sleep, have a sleep too.

Sleep

If you are not sleeping well, or find it difficult to get to sleep, try this to see just how much sleep you are actually getting. Keep a pad and pen by the bed and write down the time every 15 minutes while you are awake. This way you'll be able to tell when you fell asleep and so work out how much sleep you have actually had from the time when you woke up. Then rather than saying, 'I didn't sleep a wink last night', you will know that actually you had, for example, a total of four and three-quarter hours. It is much better for your mental health to be positive about how much sleep you actually had, rather than exaggerating and making it sound like you had none at all.

The monotony of routine

Look at your everyday life – do you feel that it is boring, repetitive and dull? Would that be an exaggeration? If not then you need to do something about it. The harsh truth is that mothering is a very repetitive job. I can't tell you how to make it less repetitive. It simply is.

However, I can give you some ideas for breaking up the monotony of mothering, and taking better care of yourself in the process. If you, like many of us, find this endless repetition brain-numbingly dull, then try asking other people to help you with those tasks, using the ideas from earlier in this chapter. Share out the workload. It's OK. Just because she is your baby doesn't mean you have to do everything for her. Let others help you, so that you can balance your daily tasks with interesting, relaxing and rewarding things. If you reduce the number of negative tasks and include more positive elements to your routine, this will help restore the balance in your life, and ultimately help you enjoy your baby.

Time for yourself

It is very important to have time for yourself so that you don't feel resentful of those around you. You have control over this. After all, it is your choice to put the washing up/cleaning/ironing higher up your priority list than your own happiness. You can decide that it doesn't all have to be done now, some can wait till later. Or someone else could do it.

So what could you do in your time for yourself that would move yourself up that priority list? You could make time each day to, for example, listen to music, paint your nails, have a bath, wash your hair, put on your make-up, read a magazine, watch a TV programme or listen to a radio programme you like, or perhaps just sit in silence. Whatever lights your fire. If it makes you feel better, then do it. It is better to start off with something small and simple so that you can actually do it – that way you will feel you have achieved something, making you feel even better. If you don't feel you can do something like this every day to start with, try it every other day or every few days at first.

Obviously some of these things require a bit of planning, and maybe someone to look after the baby, so think about working through the problem-solving guide sheet at the end of this chapter to plan how you are going to successfully get some time to yourself to do what you want with it.

Your future

The future. Those two words may be completely meaningless to you at the moment. Everything may seem hopeless right now, but you must remember that will change. You and your family do have a future. You can shape that future into something you want – or you can let the present situation, complete with your illness, continue.

You are already turning away from how your life has been recently as you are reading this book. The seeds of hope for your future are being planted. You need to water them.

Ask yourself the following questions, and answer them as honestly as you can. Note down your thoughts in the space beneath each question if you like. It will be useful for you to look back on them in the future to see if it worked out that way.

- What would you like to achieve by the baby's first birthday? This could be anything: feeling better, going back to work, being a good enough mother, not being frightened to ask for help.

- What would you like to remember about your baby's first year? Again, this could be anything: you felt better as each month went by, you allowed your mum to help you, you and your partner became closer.

The harsh truth is that you only get one chance at your baby's first year of life. If it has been rotten so far, now is the time to change it.

It is very important that on a day-to-day basis, both now and throughout the months and years to come, you should not expect too much of yourself – you can only do your best. It is essential that you ask for and get help from people you trust, and that you talk to someone you trust about how you feel, about both the ups and the downs of becoming and being a parent.

The typical pattern of recovery

Recovery from an illness like postnatal depression is gradual. Try to take life one day at a time. There will be good days and there will be bad days. Slowly but surely, once you have found and accepted practical help and emotional support that suits you, you will notice that the good days start to outnumber the bad days.

While you are recovering, try not to be too hard on yourself. Becoming a mum really is just like taking on a new job. Whether or not this is your first baby, you will be learning to cope with lots of new experiences all the time. Go easy on yourself as you will be faced with doing many new things and it is very unlikely that all will go well the first time round. If this were a new job you would probably be more forgiving to yourself. Try and remember that good enough is OK.

A gradual return to wellness is not just what is likely to happen, it is also advisable. Imagine you had broken your leg. On the day you had the plaster taken off you would not expect to be able to walk around on it as if it had never been broken. The same is true with your mind. Your brain is the part of your body that gets you round your social and emotional world. Your leg gets you round your physical world. Have respect for the fragility of your mind and the illness it is trying to overcome – or you might well end up with it back in plaster again.

Monitoring your recovery

One of the best ways to monitor your recovery is to write down your feelings, hopes and fears. Your thoughts may feel like they are whirling around your head so fast and erratically that you can't quite capture them. Not being able to think clearly is a common symptom of postnatal depression. Thoughts are easier to deal with objectively when they are written down. Some people say that it's almost as if their thoughts have become someone else's thoughts, like reading the problem page in a magazine.

Keeping a feelings diary

Many women have told me that keeping a diary of how they were feeling really helped. Your feelings diary is entirely personal to you. At first you may not want to use it every day – perhaps just write down how you feel once a week on the same day, or every few days or every other day. You don't have to go out and buy, or ask your partner to go out and buy, an actual diary. A notepad or just some scrap paper stapled or clipped together will do.

In fact, you may not want to write anything down at all. You could keep a feelings diary in your head at first, just spending a moment remembering what you were doing this time last week and comparing how you feel now with how you felt then. But it may be much easier for you to monitor your recovery over the coming weeks and months if you write something down that you can later look back at.

You may only feel like writing something down when you have had a bad day. But it will be much more helpful to write something down on your good days as well. If you focus on the good days and the positive aspects of your life, you will be more likely to feel positive about yourself and your life.

But if you have had a particularly bad day, writing down how you feel can provide you with a feeling of release. All that frustration, desperation and irritation can be poured out on a piece of paper and then, if you like, torn up or screwed up and thrown in the bin. Good riddance to bad feelings. Remember that it would be best to vent your spleen on a separate piece of paper, not in your diary, so you don't have to tear up the whole thing and throw it away! Unless you want to when you have recovered, of course . . .

The idea of a feelings diary is that you will be able to see for yourself how you are gradually recovering. The balance is being restored to include more good days and fewer bad days.

It is very important to be honest with yourself. Consider keeping the diary somewhere secure so that you know you can be absolutely frank in what you write down. If you live with your partner, let him know that you are keeping a diary, and that it is private and personal. You may want to talk to him about it, and give him a summary of your recovery, but you may not want him to read just exactly how you felt last Tuesday when he didn't do the shopping you asked for.

When looking back over your diary entries in the early days of your recovery, be careful not to become too dispirited if you see no apparent progress for a while. In time you will be able to see that balance is being restored to you and your life.

On the next few pages are two copies of the problem-solving guide sheet referred to in this chapter. If you think you might need more than two, it would be a good idea to make some copies of this guide sheet so that you can fill them in when you need to, as you try to find practical solutions to your particular problems or situations.

How to successfully solve everyday problems
guide sheet

1 *Identify what exactly the problem is.*

2 *Think about the ways you could try to solve that problem.*
If possible, think of at least three, to give you some choices.

3 *Decide which is the best way for you to try to solve that problem.*
Think about the practicalities of each choice, weighing them up
against each other and your own ability to actually do them.

4 *Attempt to solve that problem in that way.*
Think about what you will physically need to do, in what order, to give yourself the best chance of successfully solving this problem.

5 *Assess whether that action did solve that problem.*
Decide how you will know the problem is solved; you can decide this for yourself and/or ask others what they think.

6 *Praise yourself for applying the solution to the problem.*
Think about how you expected it to go – did you think it would be more or less difficult than it actually was? You know that simply doing a plan and putting it into action is something to feel proud of on its own. How will you reward yourself?

How to successfully solve everyday problems
guide sheet

1 *Identify what exactly the problem is.*

2 *Think about the ways you could try to solve that problem.*
If possible, think of at least three, to give you some choices.

3 *Decide which is the best way for you to try to solve that problem.*
Think about the practicalities of each choice, weighing them up against each other and your own ability to actually do them.

4 *Attempt to solve that problem in that way.*
Think about what you will physically need to do, in what order, to give yourself the best chance of successfully solving this problem.

5 *Assess whether that action did solve that problem.*
Decide how you will know the problem is solved; you can decide this for yourself and/or ask others what they think.

6 *Praise yourself for applying the solution to the problem.*
Think about how you expected it to go – did you think it would be more or less difficult than it actually was? You know that simply doing a plan and putting it into action is something to feel proud of on its own. How will you reward yourself?

5

Staying well

Suggestions to help you stay healthy

This chapter is about how you can look after yourself during the period of your illness. The following advice is a summary of the things talked about so far in this book plus a few extra ideas for you to consider. These ideas should help you to stay well once you begin to recover. But you don't need to wait until you are feeling depressed to follow this advice. You don't need to be a woman either. Anyone can follow these suggestions to help them stay healthy at any time.

Things to try

Take life one day at a time

Try to find the positive in things. Not everything in your life is negative all the time, even if it feels like it. Making yourself find positive aspects of your day may not be easy, but please do try, as focusing on the positive is a very simple way of helping yourself to keep feeling better. If you don't look for the positive things in your life you won't see them.

Talk to others even if you don't feel like it

You may feel that talking about your depression will just perpetuate it, and not actually solve anything. But at the very least you will have helped someone else feel that they can help you, that you trust them enough to confide in them. When we feel down we tend to feel down about everything in our life, including our relationships with loved ones, assuming they won't understand. Many women have said to me that their partner (their mothers come a close second) 'never knows what I am thinking or feeling'. Well, he's not telepathic! Are you? I know I'm not. Tell him how you feel and let him know what you think might help you (you can at least tell him what *isn't* helpful). Then at least you have given him the opportunity to show he cares for you. Just talking to him may make you feel better. Try not to push him away, hide from him or exclude him from how you feel – this won't make things better, and may mean that your relationship will be weakened by your illness, when potentially it could be strengthened.

Involve your partner or someone you are close to as much as possible

Be open about your feelings and worries. This will help your partner understand what you need. Perhaps you could look back together at your feelings diary entries to see for yourselves how much you have improved over the last few months. Remind yourself how far you have come, and how much talking to him and gaining reassurance from him has helped you. This will encourage you to continue communicating and looking after each other.

Let yourself and your partner be intimate

Even if you don't yet feel like sex, a kiss and a cuddle can be a source of great comfort and reassurance of the love you feel for each other. In your own time this can help bring about the return of full sexual desire for you both. But do be patient with yourself and with each other.

Talk to your midwife, health visitor or GP

Whatever you want to know, no question is ever too small or too silly. They are trained to help you get well and they want to help keep you well. They may even have some personal experience of postnatal depression. They, or someone they are close to, may have suffered this illness too.

Set aside time for relaxing with family and friends

You don't have to go out – stay in and ask others to come and see you. Find time to have fun. It doesn't have to be expensive; you don't have to go out for a night on the tiles. But if you do get genuine offers to babysit and money isn't too tight, then accept the help you have been offered and go out for a meal, go to the cinema, or simply visit friends. Make time to enjoy yourself with the people you love and who love you.

Take every available opportunity to rest

It is important to get some rest and relaxation each day. The relaxation techniques taught antenatally are just as useful once the baby is born. There are many types of relaxation techniques, some of which can be done anywhere at any time; you don't have to be flat on your back in a silent room. Try to learn the art of catnapping, so that you can have a small sleep while your baby does the same. Perhaps your partner can give the baby a bottle feed during the night, using expressed milk if you like.

Do some gentle exercise

Exercising is good as it can soon help you start to feel better about yourself. Local leisure centres may have classes for relaxation and exercise, such as postnatal exercise groups, aqua-natal classes or yoga, and they often have crèche facilities. They are also a good way of getting out and meeting other mothers with young babies and/or children.

If you don't feel ready to meet other mothers yet, just getting out of the house and going for a walk should help you feel better.

Eat a balanced diet

Eating properly is just as important as exercise. Mothers often are so busy looking after the needs of their baby that they forget about themselves. You may be keen to lose the weight you gained in pregnancy, and want to start dieting soon after the baby is born. My sister-in-law recently had a baby and was feeling fed up with feeling less than toned; she said that it had taken nine months for her body to produce a baby, and it would probably take another nine months to recover from it. Remember that you do need time to recover, and a good diet and exercise will help you regain your health and vitality. Try to eat little and often as this will give you a constant supply of energy – food is fuel.

Ask for help with practical jobs

Ask people you trust to help you with tasks like housework and supermarket shopping. One group of women I knew devised a plan, that the four of them would get together every Monday morning and draw lots: two would go to the supermarket and two would stay at home with the children and babies. That way the mothers all got to see each other, before and after the supermarket, the shopping got done with no tantrum-throwing (by the children), and the children and babies all got to play with each other. Do accept offers of help from people you feel comfortable with. They want to help you, and you need the help, so let them!

Find out about groups in your area and contact them

Mothers in similar situations can be an invaluable emotional and practical support to each other. Look for local postnatal support groups. These are a good way of meeting up with other mothers, exchanging information, relaxing and building up confidence about skills such as breastfeeding and baby care. Your local health visitor or midwife should know what groups there are in your area. Find out about them now if you can; although you may not feel up to going along just yet, if you find you want to in the future you will have something to look forward to.

Be honest about how you feel

At least be honest with yourself. And in groups of women with young babies and children, if you mention that you feel dreadful, like you don't know what you are doing, that you're depressed or that you can't cope, you will often find at least one other person who feels the same way. Even if there is no one who feels as bad as you do at the moment, you may find someone who has felt the same in the past, with a previous baby, or who has felt down from time to time and found a way of getting through it. The main thing is that the women there will want to help you.

There may be someone there who wants to tell the others that they feel like that too, but can't. Now that you have had the strength and courage to talk about it, you will, in all probability, have helped that mother feel better about herself for the first time in ages. She is not alone. Just like you.

Distract yourself from the more dreary repetitious side of mother-hood

Try doing something you enjoy or used to enjoy. Perhaps prepare a list now of things you would like to do, so that when you have a moment, and being a mother means that this could happen at irregular and unpredictable times, you will have some ready-made options to choose from. And depending on how much time is available, you can choose an activity from your list that fits.

It would be useful to have a mixture of passive and active distractions on your list. Passive distractions are things that take very little energy and are often initiated by someone else, for example talking to your friend on the telephone or replying to a text message. Active distractions might include deciding to go for a walk with a friend and her children and ringing them to arrange it. Be imaginative – keep adding to your list as ideas come to you, and perhaps give items a star rating: say one star for a quick fix, two stars for an hour's distraction and three for a morning or an afternoon's entertainment.

Tell yourself how well you are doing

Leave positive, encouraging notes to yourself on your noticeboard, on your fridge door, on your kettle, on your computer screen at work, on your locker door at work, on your mobile phone greeting message, in your purse, in fact wherever you are likely to see them at random times during the day. Write anything you like on your notes to yourself, about how well you are doing. It may sound mad, but little things like this can make us feel positive. They help us to remember that we are OK, that we are doing well.

Organize a daily treat, however small

Try to fit in a walk in the park, a workout, or simply a chat with friends. Remember to make time for you to maintain the balance between the negative and the positive aspects of being a mother. This can be away from your baby – you could enjoy a reflexology or aromatherapy session. Or it could be with your baby, such as attending baby massage classes, which will help strengthen the bond between you and your baby and encourage you to have some fun together.

Things to avoid

Don't be a superhero

Caring for your new baby 24 hours a day will logically mean that you need to reduce commitments in other areas of your life. You cannot have it all exactly the way you want it. Something will have to give. Perfection is something to be aspired to but don't expect to achieve it. Good enough is good enough. Make sure that you don't compromise your own health and happiness while striving for something that simply isn't possible.

Try to avoid situations that could be stressful

If something isn't going to make you feel better, don't do it. And don't feel bad about not doing it, either. You are important too. It is perfectly OK to put your own needs first once in a while, particularly if you are bright enough to realize that something will make you feel worse and so avoid doing it. I call that wisdom.

Try giving up coffee, tea, cola drinks and alcohol

All these can disrupt your ability to sleep. Having a drink containing caffeine once or twice a day will be unlikely to do you any harm, but if you are not used to it, having just one more caffeine drink than usual in a day can make you feel lousy. So too can alcohol. Try some of the numerous caffeine-free drinks available in supermarkets and health food shops nowadays: fruit teas, herbal teas, decaffeinated tea and coffee. There is also a much wider range than ever before of decaffeinated soft drinks and alcohol-free or low-alcohol alternatives. If you feel OK having the odd glass of wine, a gin and tonic, or half of lager, then go ahead.

But if you wonder whether any of these might be disturbing your sleep (and I never believed it until I tried it), don't have any of them for a few days and see for yourself if it helps you.

Don't plan to move house

Try to avoid the stress of moving house for some months after the baby is born and until after you start to feel better. This advice actually goes for anything big and disruptive that you can possibly avoid, such as you or your partner changing jobs. You will probably feel that you have got enough on your plate without anyone adding more to it, so if you can, choose not to let anyone do so. And if you can't, prepare yourself for needing extra help: ask for help and accept it. You now know those are good, healthy things to do.

Don't be too hard on yourself or your partner

Don't blame yourself or your partner for your depression. It won't help. It won't make the depression go away. Blaming yourself or others is not helpful for anyone, least of all you. Accept that life is tough at this time. Arguments about small, unimportant things will weaken your relationship when it needs to be at its strongest. Try to care for one another, not take out your frustrations on each other.

6

Supporting the depressed mother: how to help

This chapter looks at how partners, family and friends can help the woman with postnatal depression. It would be good for your partner, family and friends to read this chapter so that they understand clearly what kind of help you need. In addition, it emphasizes how important it is that they look after themselves too. They should not feel that they have to take on the role of supporter alone; it is a good idea to seek help and advice for themselves, to gather knowledge about postnatal depression so they can understand what the illness involves.

It can be difficult for partners, family and friends to understand what postnatal depression is and what they can do to help, especially if they have never encountered it before. They see their wife/daughter/best friend behaving differently, but they don't necessarily understand why this is happening. Throughout this book, I have been encouraging her to get you to read it too, and talk to you about how she feels. Thank you for reading this book; it will help. Please make sure you talk about what you have read – even if it is to disagree with what I have written! I don't care, just as long as you are talking to each other.

Living with a woman who has postnatal depression can be very difficult and frustrating. To help you through this time it might be useful for you to think of the baby's arrival as a crisis that will pass.

Do your best to be supportive, give encouragement and offer hope. Be patient and understanding. Your help at this time of crisis is absolutely invaluable. Most importantly for you, be prepared to seek help, both for her and for yourself, if you feel you need it.

Family and friends

Be reassured, there are a number of things you, as one of the depressed mother's family or circle of friends, can do to help her become and then stay well.

Do try to . . .

Sensitively ask her what she feels she needs

She will probably have a good idea of what someone might do for her to help her feel better. At the very least, she is likely to know what she doesn't want. If she is not able even to work this out at the moment, remember that as she continues to recover this will change. When you notice that she is feeling better, ask her again what she thinks she needs. It is a difficult balance to try and achieve: caring for her without irritating her. But it is important to encourage her to think about how you can help her; thinking about it will clarify for her what specific difficulties she has.

Encourage her to ask for help

Suggest that she approaches her midwife, health visitor or GP to ask for help. This is to be encouraged throughout her recovery period. If either of you has any doubts or concerns, try to arrange to see whichever one she feels she can confide in. Offer to go with her or arrange for them to come to see you at home. You could offer to be present in a supportive capacity if you think that might help her to actually get help.

Suggest she joins a support group

As mentioned earlier, exchanging experiences with people in a similar position, and realizing that you are not the only one suffering, can be an enormous relief. Again, this may not be something she feels she wants to do at first, but as things improve she may change her mind. If it is appropriate, offer to go with her.

Offer help with child care

She will probably feel that she needs to have some time away from the baby, although, she may not feel able to say this. She may feel guilty about not wishing to be with her baby all the time, and not want to let you know that. If you offer to have the baby, you remove the potential obstacle of her having to ask you, and feeling like she has to have a 'genuine' reason for asking. Wanting some time for herself is a genuine reason. When she is first recovering from her illness she may not feel able to ask for help, but may be willing to accept help that is offered and fits in with what she feels she needs.

So, as much as you can, offer to have the baby so that she can have time for herself, or for whatever other genuine reason.

Offer practical help

Offer to do the cleaning/washing/ironing while she spends some time relaxing and getting to know her baby. She may be very sensitive about this, and feel ashamed if she has let the standards of her home drop. Many women with postnatal depression have no energy to look after themselves, let alone their home, so this isn't unusual. It is important that someone else can do the cleaning/ washing/ironing while she does the relaxing and bonding. Depression usually causes a severe drop in concentration so concentrating solely on her baby, even for a short while, will be exhausting for her. But it will also probably be very rewarding.

Be patient

Please remember that depression is an illness. She cannot help suffering the symptoms that she does. Hopefully she is doing all she can for herself to move towards thinking positively and feeling better. Recovery from depression is a gradual process. Slowly but surely she will start to feel better with your support. Throughout the early months of her feeling well again, she will probably still need your help. Looking to the future, your help should prevent her becoming unwell again.

Let her express her true feelings

Please be aware that it may not be easy for you to hear what she has to say. Treat her hopes, fears and doubts seriously. Be as sympathetic as you can be. It will have taken great courage to admit these feelings to herself; saying them aloud to you will have taken even more. You may feel that you are hearing the same things again and again, and wonder if talking about it is really helping her. Some people do need to talk about things that worry them endlessly; others may not want to talk much at all. Whatever suits that person is to be encouraged. Talking about her illness a moderate amount will usually help, but if you do feel that the amount she talks about how she feels is not helping her to recover, talk about it sensitively with her. You may be able to see things she can't, as an outsider looking in, and give her new perspectives on her recovery.

Find out more about postnatal depression

She may be too ill to do this for herself, or frightened of what she may find out. Learning about her illness and depression in general will also help you to continue supporting her in a sympathetic way. Try not to slip into the age-old temptation of telling her to 'pull yourself together'. She will not appreciate it. If she could, she would. In some research I did recently, I found that most people feel that it is OK to tell yourself to pull yourself together, but not for others to tell you to do so. The implication was that the people who tell you to pull yourself together don't understand how you feel. So try not to lose your patience and blurt something out that you will both regret.

Partner and/or baby's father

You are perhaps the most pivotal person in terms of helping her to become and stay well. While this may seem very flattering, it may sometimes feel like a burden. Try to remember that she does not *want* to be a burden to you. She does not *want* to be ill. Together you can help her to become well again. Hopefully when she feels better you will feel that your relationship is stronger for the experience of surviving this difficult time.

All the suggestions in the previous section will help, in addition to the following.

Do try to . . .

Reassure her that she will get well

Frequently encourage her to believe that her illness is temporary and that in time she will get well. And as she starts to feel better, point out her progress to her. That way she knows that even if she finds herself slipping backwards at any time during her recovery, it won't last for ever, and she will feel better soon.

Reassure her of your love and support

Whether you tell each other every day that you love each other, or only on special occasions like wedding anniversaries and holidays, find a way to tell her, reassuringly, that you love her and are there for her. If you can't actually say it to her because it's something you don't feel comfortable doing, you could leave her a note, give her a great big cuddle, bring her a cup of tea in bed, or send her a text message. Whatever works for you. But do it, and do it regularly, she needs you to. Let her know that you will not abandon her. She will fear this greatly. Again if you find these things difficult to say, please find another way to show her you care.

Ensure she gets enough food and rest

Actually this goes for both of you. It may be difficult for you to check that she is eating OK if she is at home while you are at work. You could leave a prepared meal for her in the fridge the evening before, so all she has to do is zap it in the microwave. Ask her if there's anything she would really like to eat, and get it from the supermarket when you do the shopping.

Noticing if she is sleeping OK should be easier if you share a bed or a bedroom. Offer to do some of the night feeds. Perhaps once a week, when you don't have to go to work the next day, you could do all the feeds and she could have a whole night's unbroken rest. What bliss.

Encourage her to be active

Even though she might resist in the early stages of her recovery, doing something as simple as going for a short walk together will help both of you feel better. Small changes to her life that include you as her partner and your family will make it more likely that she will keep looking after herself better. For example, the whole family could go for a short walk together, or you could all eat more healthy foods more regularly and drink more water instead of caffeine or alcohol-containing drinks.

Point out how she is improving

Notice any small improvements in her well-being, and point them out to her. Praising her will reinforce the behaviour that has led to that improvement and give her the hope and courage to continue. Genuine praise for all achievements will have a massive impact on her self-esteem. But beware, if the praise is not genuine she will spot it and you could undermine her confidence further. A social worker colleague of mine once told me that the key to her success with getting people to make changes to their lives and feel better as a result of those changes was to take the following stance: if you flood a person with positive feelings and praise, then there is no room for the negative feelings. So do your best to avoid making critical comments, but consistent, genuine praise is vital as this gives her a positive structure to try and live within.

Give her a massage

Don't worry, you don't need to be an expert – most of us aren't. Try some gentle stroking of her neck, shoulders and back to start with, or you could massage her feet. Talk to each other about which bit of her body she would like to be massaged. Maybe she could return the compliment and give you a back or foot massage.

If the subject of sex has been difficult for you recently then this is a good way to break down the barriers that have grown up between you. But it is very important that if she does not want the massage to lead to anything more, like sex, you respect that. If you are aware of this and have talked about it at the outset you will know not to let yourself get carried away, and so avoid feeling let down if and when it doesn't happen. If you both know the boundaries and that you are doing this to make each other feel better, without the possibility of anything happening to disturb the trust you have between you, you will both get more from it. It should help you both to relax and restore your feelings of well-being.

Go out together as a couple

Try to arrange an outing without your baby and/or children. She may not feel this possible when she is just starting to recover, but in time you will both feel that you want to make the effort to enjoy each other's company as a couple and not simply as mum and dad. If she is resistant to your suggestions to go out together, don't force her if she isn't ready. Try not to be too offended. Because of her illness she probably doesn't feel she wants to go out with anyone at the moment, not just you. Perhaps you could ask her what she does feel up to doing at the moment and try that instead.

Look after yourself

I don't believe that postnatal depression is a gender-exclusive illness; that is, you can develop it too. It would be a good idea for you to look at the 'Suggestions to help you stay healthy' mentioned in Chapter 5. If you are following these simple steps as well, it will make it easier for her to stick to them, as she will have someone she trusts to do them with – you.

Get help if you need it at any time

Please don't keep your problems to yourselves. There are a number of organizations that can offer you advice and support. Carers UK, MIND (the National Association for Mental Health), SANE, and the Royal College of Psychiatrists all offer information about mental illness, and how to cope with living with someone who has an illness such as postnatal depression. The contact details, including websites and email addresses for these organizations can be found in Useful Addresses.

Postnatal depression threatens many things: both the mother's and father's health, their relationship with each other, their relationships with their other children and their families, their friendships and their careers, and last but certainly not least, the baby's welfare. Dealing with it on a day-to-day basis can be a huge challenge for family and friends. With support and patience from you all together, you will help the depressed mother to recover.

Useful Addresses

The following organizations will be able to offer you information, support and advice. This is just a selection of those available. Their specific role is to help you, so if you have a question just telephone them, send them an email, or have a look at their website.

Alcohol and drug addictions

Alcoholics Anonymous
If you or someone you know needs help with a drink problem, contact the Helpline:
Tel: 0845 769 7555
Website: www.alcoholics-anonymous.org.uk

Cyswllt Ceredigion Contact
A registered UK charity incorporating a Day Service that provides help, advice and support for people with drug and alcohol problems, and for their families. Also offers support to people with eating disorders. Cyswllt Ceredigion Contact consists of dedicated, specialist, trained staff.
Tel: 01970 626470
Email: office@recovery.org.uk
Website: www.recovery.org.uk

Narcotics Anonymous
A non-profit fellowship of men and women for whom drugs had become a major problem. Run by recovering addicts who meet regularly to help each other stay clean. To find your local group:
Tel: 020 7730 0009
Email: helpline@ukna.org
Website: www.ukna.org

Baby massage

Guild of Infant and Child Massage
Maintains a national and international register of professional members that is available for the general public and to other professional disciplines. To find a qualified teacher local to you:

Tel: 01889 564555
Email: enquiries@gicm.org.uk
Website: www.gicm.org.uk

International Association of Infant Massage
Coordinates and assists the work of the rapidly growing number of Certified Infant Massage Instructors, and can provide a list of qualified instructors.
Tel: 07816 289 788 (Tuesday to Thursday 9 a.m.–5 p.m.)
Email: mail@iaim.org.uk
Website: www.iaim.org.uk

Benefits, money and debt

The Maternity Alliance
A national charity working to improve rights and services for pregnant women, new parents and their families. Information about maternity benefits is available via their helpline and website.
Tel: 020 7490 7638
Email: office@maternityalliance.org.uk
Website: www.maternityalliance.org.uk

National Debtline
A helpline that provides free confidential and independent advice on how to deal with debt problems.
Tel: 0808 808 4000
Email: advice@nationaldebtline.co.uk
Website: www.nationaldebtline.co.uk

Breastfeeding

Association of Breastfeeding Mothers
Information and advice on breastfeeding and support for breastfeeding mothers.
Tel: 0870 401 7711 (24-hour helpline)
Email: counselling@abm.me.uk or info@abm.me.uk
Website: www.abm.me.uk

La Lèche League
Aims to help mothers to breastfeed through mother-to-mother support, encouragement, information and education. Also aims to promote a better understanding of breastfeeding as an important element in the healthy development of the baby and mother.

Tel: 0845 120 2918 (24-hour helpline)
Email: lllgb@wsds.co.uk
Website: www.laleche.org.uk

National Childbirth Trust (NCT)
Offers antenatal classes, befriending, coffee groups, postnatal classes, and breastfeeding counsellors. For the contact details of your local breastfeeding counsellor:
Tel: 0870 770 3236
Breastfeeding line: 0870 444 8708 (daily 8 a.m.–10 p.m.)
Email: enquiries@national-childbirth-trust.co.uk
Website: www.nctpregnancyandbabycare.com

Complementary therapies

British Acupuncture Council
The UK's main regulatory body for the practice of acupuncture by over 2,400 professionally qualified acupuncturists. To find an accupuncturist:
Tel: 020 8735 0400
Email: info@acupuncture.org.uk
Website: www.acupuncture.org.uk

British Chiropractic Association
The largest and longest-established association for chiropractors in the UK. To find a chiropractitioner local to you:
Tel: 0118 950 5950
Email: enquiries@chiropractic-uk.co.uk
Website: www.chiropractic-uk.co.uk

British Reflexology Association
Founded in 1985 to act as a representative body for reflexology practitioners and for students training in the method. To find a reflexologist:
Tel: 01886 821 207
Email: bra@britreflex.co.uk
Website: www.britreflex.co.uk

Craniosacral Therapy Association of the United Kingdom
Exists to provide support for practitioners of craniosacral therapy, to find a craniosacral practitioner local to you:

Tel: 07000 784 735
Email: office@craniosacral.co.uk
Website: www.craniosacral.co.uk

General Osteopathic Council
Includes the Osteopathic Information Service and a database for you
to find a registered osteopath local to you.
Tel: 020 7357 6655 (Monday to Friday 9 a.m.–5 p.m.)
Email: info@osteopathy.org.uk
Website: www.osteopathy.org.uk

Institute for Complementary Medicine
A registered charity formed in 1982 to provide the public with
information on complementary medicine. The ICM administers the
British Register of Complementary Practitioners (BRCP), which is a
register of professional, competent practitioners whom have all been
assessed individually, such as aromatherapists.
Tel: 020 7237 5165
Email: info@icmedicine.co.uk
Website: www.i-c-m.org.uk

Depression

Carers UK
Campaigns for the rights of carers in the UK and provides
information and advice for carers on any issue.
Tel: 020 7490 8818
Email: info@ukcarers.org
Website: www.carersonline.org.uk

MIND (National Association for Mental Health)
Information services for all matters relating to mental health in
England and Wales.
Tel: 0845 766 0163 (Monday to Friday 9.15 a.m.–4.45 p.m.)
Email: contact@mind.org.uk
Website: www.mind.org.uk

Royal College of Psychiatrists
Information about mental illness.
Tel: 020 7235 2351
Email: rcpsych@rcpsych.ac.uk
Website: www.rcpsych.ac.uk

Samaritans
A confidential listening service for any person who is suicidal or despairing.
Tel: 08457 90 90 90
Textphone: 08457 90 91 92
Email: Jo@samaritans.org
Website: www.samaritans.org.uk

SANE
Information and support to anyone coping with a mental illness. Contact the helpline:
Tel: 0845 767 8000 (daily 12 noon–2 a.m.)
Email: london@sane.org.uk; bristol@sane.org.uk; macclesfield@sane.org.uk
Website: www.sane.org.uk

Domestic violence and sexual abuse

Rape & Sexual Abuse Support Centre (RASASC)
A helpline providing information and counselling for victims of rape and sexual abuse.
Tel: 020 8683 3300 or 020 8683 3311 (counselling)
Website: www.rasasc.org.uk

Victim Support
A helpline provides information and support to victims of all reported and unreported crime, including sexual crimes, racial harassment, and domestic violence.
Tel: 0845 30 30 900
Email: contact@victimsupport.org.uk
Website: www.victimsupport.org

Women's Aid
Offers a freephone 24-hour National Domestic Violence Helpline, run in partnership by Women's Aid and Refuge.
Tel: 0808 2000 247
Email: info@womensaid.org.uk
Website: www.womensaid.org.uk

Eating disorders

Cyswllt Ceredigion Contact
A registered UK charity incorporating a Day Service that provides help, advice and support to people with eating disorders. Cyswllt Ceredigion Contact consists of dedicated, specialist, trained staff.
Tel: 01970 626470
Email: office@recovery.org.uk
Website: www.recovery.org.uk

Eating Disorders Association
Information and help on all aspects of eating disorders, including anorexia nervosa, bulimia nervosa, binge eating and other related eating disorders.
Tel: Adult helpline 0845 634 1414 (over 18 years) (Monday to Friday 8.30 a.m.–8.30 p.m., Saturdays 1 p.m.–4.30 p.m.)
Email: helpmail@edauk.com
Tel: Youthline 0845 634 7650 (up to and including 18 years) (Monday to Friday 4 p.m.–6.30 p.m., Saturdays 1 p.m.–4.30 p.m.)
Email: talkback@edauk.com
Text: 07977 493345
Website: www.edauk.com

Health and medical advice

Health Information Service
Information on all health-related subjects including where to get treatment.
Tel: 0800 66 55 44 (Monday to Friday 9 a.m.–7 p.m.)
Email: dhmail@doh.gsi.gov.uk
Website: www.nhs.uk

NHS Direct
A 24-hour nurse-led helpline providing confidential healthcare advice and information.
Tel: 0845 46 47
Email: via the website
Website: www.nhsdirect.nhs.uk

UKPPG Medication Helpline (United Kingdom Psychiatric Pharmacy Group)
Provides confidential information about prescription drugs from trained medical professionals.
Tel: 021 434 3270
Email: contact@ukppg.org.uk
Website: www.ukppg.org.uk

Lone or single parents

Gingerbread
Support for lone-parent families and women facing pregnancy on their own.
Tel: 0800 018 4318
Email: office@gingerbread.org.uk
Website: www.gingerbread.org.uk

One Parent Families
Promotes the welfare of lone parents and their children and has a free and confidential helpline.
Tel: 0800 018 5026
Email: info@oneparentfamilies.org.uk
Website: www.oneparentfamilies.org.uk

Parenting and family life

CRY-SIS
Support for parents whose children cry excessively, or have sleep problems or behaviour difficulties.
Tel: 020 7404 5011 (daily 9 a.m.–10 p.m.)
Email: info@cry-sis.org.uk
Website: www.cry-sis.com

Home-Start
Schemes provide trained volunteers who offer support, friendship and practical help to families with young children in the family's own home. For the contact details of your local scheme:
Tel: 08000 68 63 68
Email: info@home-start.org.uk
Website: www.home-start.org.uk

Parentline Plus
A UK registered charity that offers support to anyone parenting a child – the child's parents, step-parents, grandparents and foster-parents, including a confidential freephone helpline for anyone caring for children.
Tel: 0808 800 2222
Textphone: 0800 783 6783
Email: contact@parentlineplus.org.uk
Website: www.parentlineplus.org.uk

Postnatal depression

Association for Postnatal Illness
Information and support for women suffering from postnatal depression.
Tel: 020 7386 0868
Email: info@apni.org
Website: www.apni.org

Depression Alliance
Specifically DAPeND, the Depression Alliance Helpline for anyone affected by depression associated with childbirth.
DAPeND Helpline: 0845 120 3746
Tel: 0845 123 23 20 (Monday to Friday 10 a.m.–5 p.m.)
Email: via website
Website: www.depressionalliance.org

MAMA (Meet A Mum Association)
Support for mothers with postnatal depression. For information on support groups:
Tel: 0845 120 3746 (PND helpline, Monday to Friday 7 p.m.–10 p.m.)
Email: meet-a-mum.assoc@btinternet.com
Website: www.mama.co.uk

Pregnancy and birth

Birth Choice UK
Information on birth options and where to have your baby.
Email: feedback@BirthChoiceUK.com
Website: www.birthchoiceuk.com

Birth Crisis Network
The website gives details of phone numbers that women can ring if they want to talk about a traumatic birth. They do not give advice but offer reflective listening.
Email: birthcrisis@sheilakitzinger.com
Website: www.sheilakitzinger.com

National Childbirth Trust (NCT)
Offers antenatal classes, befriending, coffee groups, postnatal classes, and breastfeeding counsellors. For information about your local branch:
Tel: 0870 990 8040
Email: enquiries@national-childbirth-trust.co.uk
Website: www.nctpregnancyandbabycare.com

Premature babies

BabyCentre
Offers a hands-on guide to pregnancy, birth and life providing information, support and guidance during pregnancy and about bringing up a baby or toddler, including premature babies.
Email: uk_feedback@babycentre.co.uk
Website: www.babycentre.co.uk

Bliss
A premature baby charity that offers parental support and an advice network to the families of babies who need special or intensive care.
Tel: 0500 618140 (Monday to Friday 10 a.m.–5 p.m.)
Email: information@bliss.org.uk
Website: www.bliss.org.uk

Social activities and exercise

Leisure Centres
Your local leisure centre may run antenatal and postnatal exercise groups, yoga classes, aqua-aerobics classes or parent-and-toddler swimming sessions. For more details contact your local County Council Service Shop. The telephone number for your local council will be in the phone book, or you could look them up on:
Website: www.accessentertainment.co.uk/Leisure/index.htm

Playgroups, childminders, childcare and pre-school education
For information on what services are available in your area:
Tel: 08000 96 02 96
Email: via the website
Website: www.childcarelink.gov.uk

Stillbirth and miscarriage

Babyloss
Resources and support for bereaved parents who have suffered
pregnancy loss through miscarriage, ectopic pregnancy, intra-uterine
death, stillbirth or neonatal death.
Email: support@babyloss.com
Website: www.babyloss.com

SANDS (Stillbirth and Neonatal Death Society)
Works to support bereaved parents, and to press for improvements in
care during pregnancy and when a baby has died. Contact the
helpline on:
Tel: 020 7436 5881 (Monday to Friday 10 a.m.– 3 p.m.)
Email: support@uk-sands.org
Website: www.uk-sands.org

Therapy and counselling

British Association for Behavioural and Cognitive Psychotherapies
Provides a directory of registered therapists for £2.00 including
postage.
Tel: 01254 875277
Email: babcp@babcp.com
Website: www.babcp.com

British Association for Counselling and Psychotherapy
Information and advice on all matters related to counselling. They
can send you a list of accredited counsellors in your local area.
Tel: 0870 443 5252
Email: bacp@bacp.co.uk
Website: www.bacp.co.uk

CRUSE Bereavement Care
Information and advice for people who have been affected by the death of a loved one.
Tel: 0870 167 1677 (Monday to Friday 9.30 a.m.–5 p.m.)
Email: helpline@crusebereavementcare.org.uk
Website: www.crusebereavementcare.org.uk

PACE
Counselling, mental health advocacy and group work for lesbians and gay men.
Tel: 020 7700 1323 (Monday to Friday 9 a.m.–5 p.m.)
Email: info@pacehealth.org.uk
Website: www.pacehealth.org.uk

Relate
Counselling service for couples experiencing problems with their relationship. For information about your local branch:
Tel: 0845 456 1310
Email: enquiries@relate.org.uk
Website: www.relate.org.uk

Twins and multiple births

Multiple Births Foundation
An independent charity based at Queen Charlotte's and Chelsea Hospital in west London. Aims to improve the care and support of multiple birth families.

TAMBA Twinline
A national, confidential, support, listening and information service for all parents of twins, triplets or more.
Tel: 0800 138 0509 (weekdays 7 p.m.–11 p.m., weekends 10 a.m.–11 p.m.)
Email: enquiries@tamba.org.uk
Website: www.tamba.org.uk
Telephone: 020 8383 3519
Email: info@multiplebirths.org.uk
Website: www.multiplebirths.org.uk

Further Reading

By the same author:

Wheatley, Dr Sandra L., *Nine Women, Nine Months, Nine Lives*, Potent, 2001.
(ISBN 0–9540012–0–6)
Read the first chapter online at www.potent.uk.com
Freephone order line: 0800 996 1244
For all those having (or recently having had) their first child. This book contains the actual and varied experiences of nine women. From the moment they saw the positive line on the pregnancy test up until their child's first birthday, their new lives and how they feel about them, as they tell them, are presented.

Wheatley, Dr Sandra L., *Helping New Mothers to Help Themselves*, Potent, 2004
(ISBN 0–9540012–1–4)
This information pack has been written for health professionals, such as health visitors and midwives, who work with women who have antenatal or postnatal depression. It includes the 'Four-Weekly Wheatley' self-assessment questionnaire and is available on CD. It contains a series of structured visits with sufficiently detailed information sheets for the health professional to competently work through with a depressed woman various topics such as controlling negative thinking, successful problem-solving, and confidently seeking and accepting help, all of which are known to aid recovery from depression. The information pack can be tailored to work with individual women and groups of women. Training in the implementation of the information pack for teams of health professionals is available by the author via info@potent.uk.com.

The following books are arranged in alphabetical order of the author's surname, not in any order of preference. All these books are interesting and useful. If you are not sure whether you want to buy any of them, you could ask your local library if they have a copy or would order one for you to borrow.

Dalton, Katharina, *Depression After Childbirth: How to Recognize, Treat, and Prevent Postnatal Depression*, Oxford Paperbacks, 1980. (ISBN 0–19–263277–9)
The text treats postnatal depression as a hormonal rather than psychological illness. Included are chapters on hormone therapy, careers, motherhood, coping with stress, a look at the roles that partners play and the effect the illness has upon them and a chapter on maternal behaviour in animals.

Figes, Kate, *Life After Birth: What Even Your Friends Won't Tell You About Motherhood*, Viking, 1998.
(ISBN 0–670–86600–8)
Takes a hard-hitting look at the reality of becoming a mother, covering the physical, emotional, social and sexual aspects. This book sets out to dispel the myths surrounding motherhood and to address the varied needs of contemporary women facing motherhood.

Gilbert, Paul, *Overcoming Depression: A Self-help Guide Using Cognitive Behavioural Techniques*, Constable and Robinson, 2000. (ISBN 1–84119–125–6)
'A self-help manual full of step-by-step suggestions, case examples and practical ideas for gaining control over depression and low mood.' Included are chapters to help understand depression and its causes, and to help learn how to cope with depression and its various symptoms. It also contains a complete self-help programme with monitoring sheets.

Iovine, Vicki, *The Best Friend's Guide to Surviving the First Year of Motherhood*, Bloomsbury, 1999.
(ISBN 0–7475–3648–1)
The author of the *Girlfriend's Guide to Pregnancy* brings a mother's wisdom and a girlfriend's candour to a guide to motherhood. Readers will learn about baby euphoria, postpartum mood swings, salvaging one's sex life and fitting into that favourite pair of jeans.

Kitzinger, Sheila, *The Year After Childbirth: Surviving and Enjoying the First Year of Motherhood*, Oxford Paperbacks, 1994. (ISBN 0–19–286165–4)

Practical information and advice on nutrition, exercise and emotional well-being to guide new mothers through the turbulent first year after childbirth.

Shaw, Fiona, *Out of Me: The Story of a Postnatal Breakdown*, Virago Press, 2001.
(ISBN 1–86049–857–4)
Details Fiona Shaw's descent into chronic postnatal depression. Her reason for writing the book is intrinsically connected to her desire to fill in memory gaps, having received electro-convulsive therapy (ECT) as part of her treatment. Fiona wrote the book as a testimony to her illness and as her own triumph into motherhood.

Welford, Heather, *The National Childbirth Trust Book of Postnatal Depression: Helping You Through a Difficult Time*, HarperCollins, 1998.
(ISBN 0–7225–3605–4)
'This sympathetic book will answer your questions and help you seek support from those who can help.' It covers when and why PND can occur, how to ask for help, treatments available, helping your baby through a traumatic time, and advice for partner, family and friends.

Index